A Manual of Dermatology

Second Edition

DONALD M. PILLSBURY,

M.A., M.D., D.Sc. (Hon. Nebr.), F.A.C.P.
Emeritus Professor and Former Chairman,
Department of Dermatology,
School of Medicine, University of Pennsylvania;
Colonel M.C., AUS (ret.)

CHARLES L. HEATON,

M.D., M.A. (Hon. Penna.), F.A.C.P.
Associate Professor, Department of Dermatology,
College of Medicine, University of Cincinnati;
formerly Associate Professor,
Department of Dermatology,
School of Medicine, University of Pennsylvania

1980
W. B. SAUNDERS COMPANY   Philadelphia   London   Toronto

W. B. Saunders Company: West Washington Square
Philadelphia, PA   19105

1 St. Anne's Road
Eastbourne, East Sussex BN21 3UN, England

1 Goldthorne Avenue
Toronto, Ontario M8Z 5T9, Canada

Library of Congress Cataloging in Publication Data

Pillsbury, Donald Marion, 1902–

A manual of dermatology.

Includes bibliographical references.

1. Dermatology.   I. Heaton, Charles L., joint author.
  II. Title. [DNLM: 1. Skin diseases. WR140.3 P642m]

RL71.P66 1980   616.5   79–3927

ISBN 0–7216–7242–6

A Manual of Dermatology   ISBN   0-7216-7242-6

Last digit is the print number: 9   8   7   6   5   4   3   2   1

TO THE MEMORY OF
PHILADELPHIA GENERAL HOSPITAL
"OLD BLOCKLEY"
1732–1977

Preface

The primary purpose of this manual is to guide the student and the practitioner in the diagnosis and management of the skin diseases most likely to be encountered in primary care medicine. In varying detail, it addresses problems of initial assessment, simple therapy and determination of the need for further study, in perhaps 90 per cent of the common dermatoses. This edition also includes brief descriptions of less common diseases that may deserve differential consideration, and it offers an expanded chapter on cutaneous signs of systemic disease.

The second edition of *A Manual of Dermatology* is actually the fifth in a line of small and large volumes dealing with diseases affecting the skin. All of these have had gratifying acceptance. Possibly the most successful appeared in 1942 as a "war manual" designed to give help and guidance to medical officers who had no experience in dermatology and who were suddenly faced with responsibility for the care of large numbers of patients with common and uncommon skin diseases. Co-authors of that volume were Doctors Marion B. Sulzberger, Clarence S. Livingood and Donald M. Pillsbury.

Physicians in 1942 were severely handicapped by a paucity of safe and effective treatments and by a plethora of potentially harmful ones. It sometimes appeared that as many patients were harmed as were helped. When sulfonamides, antihistamines, antibiotics and corticosteroids made their clinical appearance in the 1940's and 1950's, the face of dermatologic therapy changed dramatically. Elements of risk remained, but the patient's lot was greatly improved. The past decade has been marked principally by increased sophistication of diagnostic methods, some significant advances in treatment and better understanding of the genesis of a considerable number of diseases through basic research. This current edition demonstrates, it is hoped, the major advances in the diagnosis and treatment of dermatologic diseases over the past decade.

We owe a debt to authors of other volumes, particularly to Doctors Samuel Moschella and Harry Hurley for *Dermatology,* a comprehensive, multi-authored, two-volume work (1976); to Doctors Sulzberger and Livingood as mentioned above; and to Doctors Walter B. Shelley and Albert M.

Kligman for *Dermatology* (1956) and a *Manual of Cutaneous Medicine* (1961). All of these colleagues have been sources of knowledge and stimulation at various times through many years, and we have been privileged to receive intellectual sustenance from them in abundant measure.

DMP
CLH

Acknowledgments

The chapters on basic principles of anatomy and physiology have been derived largely from *A Manual of Cutaneous Medicine* (Pillsbury, D. M., Shelley, W. B., and Kligman, A. M., W. B. Saunders Company, Philadelphia, 1961).

It will be immediately apparent that pictures, mostly in color, constitute a major part of this volume. With a few exceptions, these are from the collections of the departments of dermatology of the University of Pennsylvania and University of Miami Schools of Medicine, as listed below. We are greatly indebted to Dr. Harvey Blank for permission to use the latter collection. Comprehensive collections of this type require the efforts of many individuals through the years, and although those individuals are largely nameless here, our thanks are due to them. Mr. Edward Glifort took the photographs at the University of Pennsylvania, and Mr. William Atkinson at the University of Miami. We are also indebted to Mr. Evaristo L. Giglio, photographer at the University of Cincinnati Medical Center.

The authors gratefully acknowledge the authorship of the section on phototherapy in Chapter 14 by Kays H. Kaidbey, M.D., Department of Dermatology, School of Medicine, University of Pennsylvania.

And as has been the case on several occasions in the past thirty-six years, we are indebted to our publishers for encouragement and advice and for their superlative efficiency.

Photo Credits

Figures 1–1 to 2–3 are taken from *A Manual of Cutaneous Medicine* (Pillsbury, D. M., Shelley, W. B., and Kligman, A. M., W. B. Saunders Company, Philadelphia, 1961).

The following figures are included through the kind permission of Dr. Harvey Blank, Chairman, Department of Dermatology, University of Miami, School of Medicine: 4–5, 4–13, 5–10, 5–26, 6–5, 6–6, 6–7, 6–8, 6–16, 6–17, 6–18, 6–19, 6–24, 6–25, 6–26, 7–16, 7–17, 7–18, 7–19, 7–20, 7–21, 7–22, 7–23, 10–7, 16–2, 16–3, 17–10, 17–11, 17–12, 19–1, 19–2, 19–3.

Figures 18–9 to 18–12 are reproduced with permission from *Diseases of the Skin in Children and Adolescents* (Korting, G. W., W. B. Saunders Company, Philadelphia, 1970).

Figure 13–34 is included through the kind permission of Robert I. Rudolph, M.D., of Reading, Pennsylvania.

Figures 5–14, 5–19, 6–10, 9–10, and 18–4 are included through the kind permission of George W. Hambrick, Jr., M.D., Chairman, Department of Dermatology, College of Medicine, University of Cincinnati.

Contents

Anatomic, Physiologic and Chemical Factors in Diseases of the Skin

GENERAL CONSIDERATIONS

The main function of skin is to protect the tissues that it encloses. It is a vital shield against the shifting physical and chemical stresses of the environment. It fulfills its role to the extent that outside changes are not transmitted inward to upset internal equilibria. It is an insulator, not an organ of exchange. The physical purposes it serves are essential to life. These are:

1. *Protection* against trauma, including mechanical, thermal, chemical and radiant.

2. *Impermeability.* Very few substances go through the skin with ease. It seals man off from his complex chemical environment.

3. *Heat regulation.* Eccrine sweating produces an efficient means of losing heat so that the body temperature does not rise under heat stress or during vigorous physical exertion. Rich plexuses of fine blood vessels aid in the conservation or dissipation of heat, according to need.

4. *Touch, pain, heat* and *cold* are registered through the nerves that permeate the skin. The skin is an organ of perception par excellence. To some extent it is also an organ of expression, betraying strong feelings such as shame (blushing), anger (redness), fear (blanching) and anxiety (sweating).

The skin is stratified into three layers, from outward to within as follows:

1. The *epidermis*, a paper-thin cellular membrane

2. The *corium*, a dense connective tissue layer, mostly noncellular

3. The *subcutaneous tissue*, a thick layer that stores fat and acts as a cushion

With evolutionary progress, the skin has become increasingly complex and diversified. From the pluripotential epidermis in fetal life comes the complement of structures known as the adnexal or epidermal appendages: (1) eccrine sweat glands, (2) apocrine glands, (3) hair follicles, (4)

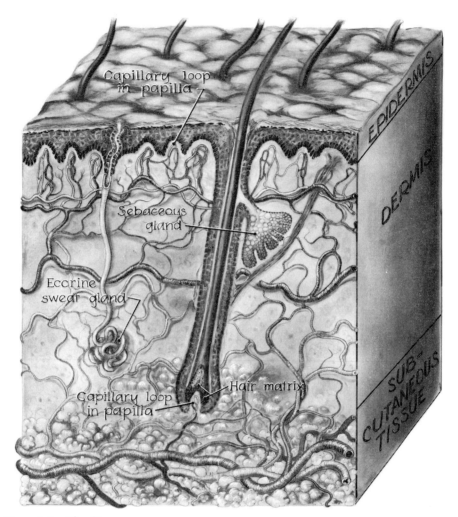

Figure 1–1. The skin

The stratified organization of the skin. The top layer, the epidermis, is thin but solidly cellular in contrast to the much thicker and largely fibrous corium which mainly acts as a support for the appendages, vessels and nerves. The hair is the deepest epidermal appendage, extending down to the subcutaneous tissue 3 to 5 mm. below the surface. Just as the hair papilla is an invagination of connective tissue into the cellular hair matrix, so the papillae of the upper corium extend upward as connective tissue intrusions into the epidermis. Each papilla has a single capillary loop which nourishes the "cap" of epithelial cells overlying it. (There are no blood vessels in the epidermis or hair matrix.) Note that eccrine sweat is delivered directly to the surface, but sebum empties into the upper part of the follicle.

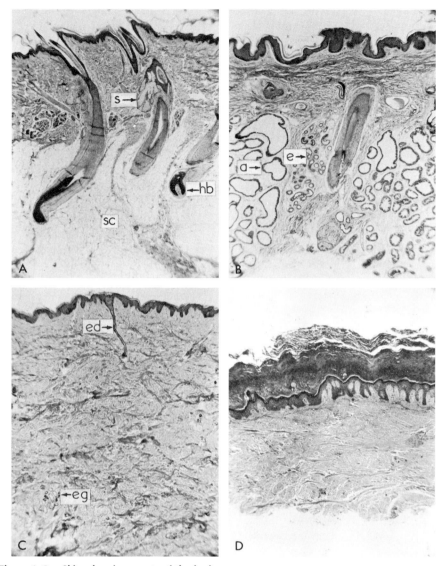

Figure 1–2. Skin of various parts of the body

Microscopic sections of skin in different parts of body. Although the skin is a single organ, different areas have peculiar anatomic and physiologic characteristics which endow them with individual attributes. No other body organ is more diversified.

These four photographs are taken at the same magnification. It is obvious that the *differences* are more marked than the *similarities* of these various skin areas.

A. Scalp. Note numerous deeply situated hair follicles (s, sebaceous glands; sc, subcutaneous tissue; hb, hair bulb). The corium is relatively thin.

B. Axilla. Excretory glands are concentrated here (a, apocrine glands; e, eccrine glands).

C. Glabrous skin of back. Note how thick the corium is; the subcutaneous tissue is too deep to be shown in toto (ed, eccrine duct; eg, eccrine gland). Appendages are not prominent in this region.

D. Palm. The stratum corneum is strikingly thick. There are no hair follicles or sebaceous glands. Eccrine glands, however, are present.

nails and (5) sebaceous glands. Ordinarily, these are not replaceable if completely lost in postnatal life. Together they make up the cutaneous epithelial system. These cells retain certain potentialities in common, remembering, as it were, their common origin.

Anatomically and physiologically the skin differs vastly in different regions. It is a genus, not a species. Each region shows the species variation to meet special stresses. Presumably, the anatomic peculiarities of diverse regions such as the soles, ear lobes, eyelids, scrotum, axillae and back are to some measure designed as adaptations. These regions vary in thickness and looseness and in the kinds and quantities of appendages they contain. These variations are the basis for (1) the localization of many disorders to special areas and (2) the distribution of certain eruptions in a characteristic pattern. The variable way in which the skin of different areas reacts to different stresses can hardly be overemphasized. It is hazardous to generalize about "skin." Dermatologic expertness requires intimate knowledge of the special propensity of each region for particular types of reactions and disorders.

The skin is traversed by furrows and ridges that make varied patterns in different regions. The whorls made by the furrows on the finger tips are an absolute signature for each person, making everyone completely individualistic in respect to his fingerprint.

Langer's lines are nonvisible cleavage planes whose distribution has been mapped out for every region of the body. Their existence is demonstrated by the simple act of puncturing the skin. A slit rather than a hole results. When possible, surgical incisions should follow these lines.

Sometimes it is forgotten that the skin is part of the body and that it is more than a shell preventing the contents from leaking out. Organ systems, such as cardiovascular, neurologic and connective tissue, have large outposts in the skin, and many systemic disorders involve the skin as well as other organs. Indeed, a skin lesion is often the first diagnostic clue to a more generalized process. More and more diseases, at first thought to be purely cutaneous, are now known to have systemic counterparts. A relatively inconspicuous lesion may resolve a large clinical puzzle. Internal derangements are often reflected in the mirror of the skin.

THE EPIDERMIS

The epidermis is a thin, totally cellular membrane devoid of lymphatics, blood vessels and connective tissue. It is parasitic on the corium, deriving its nourishment from rich capillary plexuses therein. Inflammatory processes in the dermis will, therefore, almost inevitably alter the epidermis pathologically. Since the epidermis is the surface layer of the skin, these epidermal changes are conspicuous. It is no wonder that the changes of blistering, scaling, thickening and discoloration figure heavily

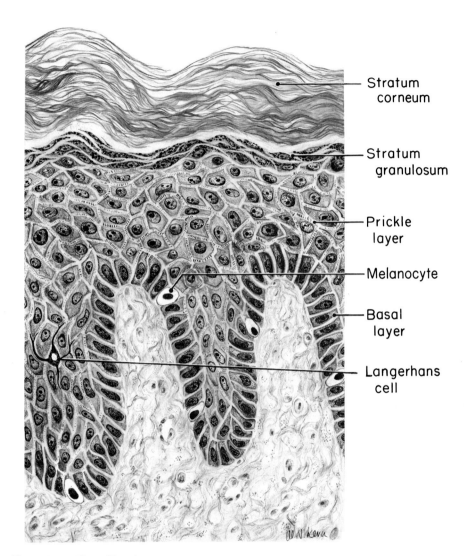

Stratum
corneum

Stratum
granulosum

Prickle
layer

Melanocyte

Basal
layer

Langerhans
cell

Figure 1–3.   The epidermis

The epidermis is stratified. The outer horny layer is dead and made up of cells which are keratinized (the cellular composition of the stratum corneum is not ordinarily evident). The basal or
lowermost layer contains the stem or mother cells from which all the other cells ultimately derive.
The melanocytes are in the basal layer and frequently look like "clear" cells. The "prickles" are
processing artifacts that represent the attachment points (desmosomes) between epithelial cells.
Langerhans cells are phagocytic, and play an important role in antigen transport between the skin
surface and regional lymph nodes.

in the description of skin disease. Functionally, the epidermis cannot be considered apart from the substrate on which it rests.

The epidermis consists of two main layers:

1. The *stratum malpighii* or *germinativum* (the living epidermis)

2. The *stratum corneum* or *horny layer* (the dead end product of epidermis)

The cells in the basal layer are the parents of all the other cells in the epidermis. These divide continuously, providing for a steady increase in the cellular population. The daughter cells are displaced outward by the steady stream of younger cells. In their journey, they progressively flatten, shrink, lose their nuclei and sojourn a short while as horny cells in the stratum corneum before being sloughed off. Probably 3 to 4 weeks are required for a basal cell to complete its life history before it is lost at the surface, even longer in thick skin. The epidermis is, thus, constantly renewing itself; cells die at the same rate at which they are born. The normal desquamation of horny cells is a microscopic process; however, in pathologic states, the cells stick together to form flakes or scales, always a sign of epidermal damage.

The epidermis is a trinary system. It contains three distinct cell types: the *keratinocyte*, which makes keratin and is responsible for the many special protective properties of the epidermis; the *melanocyte*, which makes melanin for protective pigmentation; and the *Langerhans cell*, which is responsible for phagocytosis and plays an important role in antigen transport between the surface of the epidermis and regional lymph nodes.

The Prickle Cell Layer

Just above the basal layer is the *prickle layer*, so called because the keratinocytes seem to be connected by numerous prickles. Formerly, these were thought to represent connecting bridges through which the cytoplasm of adjacent cells was continuous. The electron microscope has corrected this idea. The prickles are merely oppositely placed, rod-shaped thickenings of adjacent cell walls. The cells are glued tightly together at these points. They invariably disappear when the cohesion of epidermal cells is disrupted by blister formation. Numerous microscopic fibrils, tonofilaments, are moored at each prickle. These sweep out in various directions and attach to other prickles around the cell wall. These internal lashings, crisscrossing the cytoplasm like ropes tied at opposite ends to the cell wall, provide great physical stability. Despite its thinness, the epidermis has the toughness its external position demands. Moreover, the tonofilaments themselves are made up of a durable fibrous protein, keratin in an incomplete form. When these are destroyed, the cell tends to fall apart and separate from its neighbors. Tonofilaments and prickles are essential for keeping the epidermis intact.

The Keratinization Cycle

Keratinocytes are quite sensitive to changing stresses, whether these arise externally or within the skin. Even so minor a trauma as stripping the surface with cellophane tape a few times leads to cell enlargement and a burst of mitotic activity. Scratching alone may greatly thicken the epidermis. The health of the epidermis is dependent on the general health of the body.

The *stratum corneum, or horny layer,* is really the excretion product of the epidermis. It is a layer of interdigitated, dead, flattened, cornified cells. By casting off its own cells, the epidermis qualifies as a holocrine gland. Except for the palms and soles, the horny layer is considerably thinner than the living epidermis, but the number of cell layers is not necessarily less. Despite its thinness and unsubstantial bulk, its protective capacity is great. Its molecular brickwork, keratin, is one of the toughest of fibrous proteins; the stratum corneum is to the skin what the bark is to the tree.

The *transitional zone* between the living and dead layers of the epidermis just at the base of the stratum corneum has long been held to serve as a *barrier to penetration.* This may be an oversimplification, since the stratum corneum itself is at least a partial barrier. Not only are external substances unable to pass through the barrier, but water loss to the outside is restrained. There is about 70 per cent of water in the epidermis as compared to about 15 per cent in the horny layer. The amount of water in the stratum corneum is, to a large extent, influenced by external factors, such as temperature, relative humidity and air movements. When the atmosphere is extremely dry, especially in cold weather, the stratum corneum loses water at a rate faster than it can be replaced from below, and symptoms of chapping result. The horny layer becomes brittle and hard when its water content falls below 10 per cent. The skin looks dry and scaly. Fortunately, the horny layer is quite hygroscopic and holds on to water avidly. During bathing, the swelling and whitish wrinkling of the palms and soles are due to water absorption by the thick horny layer. The hygroscopicity of horny substance is one of its most important properties, without which it could scarcely function as a protective membrane. When its water content falls below a certain critical level, the interdigitated arrangement and close packing of the overlapping cells is disrupted; the resultant fissures and cracks expose the underlying epidermis to physical and chemical trauma, and a sequence of damaging events is initiated.

It is now appreciated that *dry skin is due not to lack of grease but rather to lack of water.* If a piece of callus is allowed to dry out, it becomes hard and brittle. Immersing it in grease will not make it flexible and soft. In water, however, it soon becomes supple and pliable. Therapeutically, dry skin is improved by water soaking followed by an application of hydrophobic grease to cut down water loss. This is only partly effective and does not correct the basic defect, which derives from an epidermal abnor-

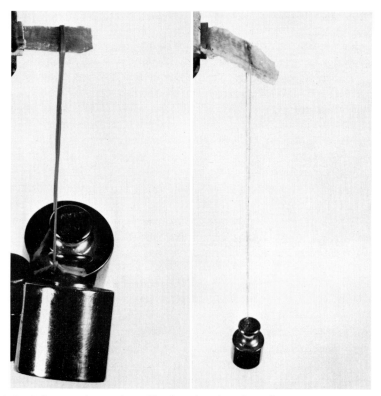

Figure 1–4. Influence of water in making keratin soft and supple

On the left is a piece of callus which has been allowed to dry out completely. Three 100 gram weights fail to bend it. After immersion in water, a ten gram weight will bend the now pliable piece of keratin.

mality. Whatever other effects they may have, fat solvents such as ether remove some substance from horny tissue, which lowers its hydrophilic capacity; therefore, they are harmful. The skin oils not only lubricate the skin but also have the important function of forming emulsions with water, thus retarding water loss. Moreover, through repeated soap and water washing, with its attendant swelling and shrinking of horn, the cellular architecture of the stratum corneum is disturbed. The surface then becomes rough and scaly. Thus, physical disorganization of the normal cellular pattern of the stratum corneum can be an accessory factor in weakening its protective capacity. It should always be remembered that clinical evidence of an abnormal stratum corneum is most often a retrospective sign of a prior injury to the underlying epidermis. Scaling of some degree is almost inevitable if epidermal cells are injured. Accordingly, many chemicals that are thought to defat or degrade horny substance produce rough skin by actually damaging the viable keratinocytes, not the dead end product.

KERATINIZATION

Keratinization may be defined in both anatomic and chemical terms. The latter refers to the synthesis of keratin, the fibrous protein that is the chief metabolic end product of epidermal cells. In anatomic terms, keratinization means the transformation of basal cells into horny cells, with all the accompanying physical changes. Tradition endorses this latter, more general, usage. Keratin is a large protein molecule made up of long amino acid chains stabilized by strong disulfide cross linkages, as well as by hydrogen and salt bonds. These cross links prevent the chains from slipping past each other. Fibrous proteins are tough, protective substances, and close packing of the cross-linked chains gives great resistance and resilience. Stability is further enhanced by the chains being wrapped around each other in a spiral arrangement. This mechanical scheme is utilized in other types of fibers in which toughness is required, as in muscle and collagen. In fact, keratin may be thought of as a muscle fiber without autocontractility. It forms the backbone of horny cells.

The formation of horny cells is so conspicuous and dominant a process that it is easy to forget that the stratum corneum is much more than keratin. Indeed, it is a kind of graveyard for all the products that are cast off during the continuous death of the epidermal cells. The nuclear and cytoplasmic constituents of epidermal cells probably are degraded and "excreted" passively into the stratum corneum. These are by-products of keratinization but not necessarily useless waste products. Included among them are water-soluble proteins, amino acids, sugars, uric acid, urea, cholesterol and minerals, the entire biochemical equipment of once living cells. After thorough extraction of horny structures with lipid solvents and water, their water-holding capacity is greatly diminished, probably through removal of certain hygroscopic components. A similar action perhaps partially accounts for the deleterious effect of repeated washing, especially with certain detergents. Such extracted horn stays brittle even though wetted. The "by-products" of cellular decomposition serve as buffers, emulsifiers, lubricants and the like to maintain the integrity of the surface. Although most of the surface fat comes from the sebaceous glands, dying epidermal cells contribute their share, the so-called horn fat. Keratin is the one substance made by epidermal cells that is not subject to decomposition by proteolytic enzymes or by microorganisms. It accumulates precisely because it is "indigestible."

In histologic sections, horny cells seem to form suddenly in the upper, moribund zone of the epidermis. This anatomic appearance is deceptive, for dying cells can scarcely have any synthetic ability. Indeed, the manufacture of keratin is almost complete in the basal layers, merely requiring some later stabilization to become a finished product. A protein with the characteristics of incomplete keratin, tonofibrin, has been isolated from epidermis. Tonofilaments are probably its anatomic substrate. This keratin precursor is later solidified in the upper epidermis by probable combination with a sulfur-containing globular protein. Keratin synthesis is thus a two-stage process. The final stage is one of sulfur enrichment, probably to form the all-important disulfide linkages that confer mechanical strength. In hair and nails, the fully formed keratin contains a great deal more disulfide sulfur than is presumably present in the matrix from which these structures spring. Hair and nails are classified as "hard" keratin, in contrast to the "soft" keratin of the stratum corneum. Horny cells containing hard keratin are packed tightly together into a homogeneous mass and do not desquamate, as do soft keratin cells. Hard keratinous structures, therefore, elongate indefinitely. The greater strength and toughness of hard keratin is attributable to its much higher disulfide content.

Keratin is usually thought of as a water-insoluble protein that is fairly resistant to dilute alkalies, strong acids and organic solvents. This is probably true of "hard" keratins. Soft keratins appear to contain about 20 per cent of a water-soluble protein that has the electrophoretic characteristics of keratin. This is possibly the precursor form, which persists unchanged. Keratin is somehow woven into the cell wall of cornified cells. Even after a strong alkaline extraction that dissolves keratin, fragments of cell walls remain, indicating the remarkable durability of the cell unit.

The process of keratin synthesis cannot be separated from multiplication of epidermal cells. More frequent divisions mean a larger quantity of keratin per unit of time. Keratin is really a holocrine "secretion." As long as cells of the stratum corneum slough off at the same rate at which they are formed, the thickness of the horny layer remains the same. An increased horny layer may mean either an increased rate of cellular division, as is characteristic of chronic inflammatory conditions, or failure of the horny cells to separate, as in ichthyosis.

Clinicians have fallen into the habit of classifying scaling or hyperkeratotic conditions as disorders of keratinization. This may be clinically convenient but does not signify an actual defect in the synthesis of keratin. In psoriasis, for instance, the keratin seems to be normal, but the water-soluble components derived from psoriatic scales are not. The confusion results from not distinguishing between the anatomic and chemical meanings of the term keratinization. It is emphasized that inflammatory conditions of the corium and epidermis invariably lead to an abnormal scaling or hyperkeratotic appearance of the stratum corneum. The primary damage, in short, is not in the horny layer.

Keratin may be readily stretched in the direction of the long axes of the molecular chains. A wet hair, for instance, can be drawn out to about one and a half times its length. During drying, the stabilizing cross linkages will pull the stretched fibers back to their original length. By chemically breaking the cross linkages after stretching the hair and reestablishing them in new positions, the extended hair may be permanently "set" in ways deemed cosmetically pleasing.

Keratinolytic agents dissolve keratin. Strong alkalies are the most potent examples. Digestion of hair, scales and nails in 10 per cent potassium hydroxide solution is the classic means of visualizing ringworm fungi. Barium sulfide creams completely dissolve hair and are thus useful as depilatories. These alkalies attack the disulfide cross linkages so that the molecular grid falls apart. In addition, the protein chains are hydrolyzed into their component amino acids. Certain alkaline reducing agents, particularly thioglycolate salts, enjoy a wide popularity as permanent cold wave sets for home use. Through controlled rupturing of disulfide bonds the hair may be stretched and molded to the desired wave. To "set" the hair, oxidizing agents are applied that re-establish the stabilizing cross links in new positions. These manipulations are a kind of chemical weaving.

Weaker keratolytic agents are widely used in clinical practice because their damaging effect is less. These include phenol, resorcinol, salicylic acid and urea. They cannot completely dissolve keratin, but by breaking hydrogen bonds, which serve as weaker cross links between protein chains, a modest degree of keratinolysis is achieved. The therapeutic effect of the agents is probably unrelated to their keratinolytic action.

HAIR

Hair is made up of tightly fused horny cells of the hard keratin variety. Because sebaceous glands are invariably associated with the hair-bearing follicles, this appendageal unit is called the pilosebaceous apparatus. It originates from the epidermis at about the third month of fetal life. After birth, the epidermis cannot generate new follicles; hence, loss by disease or trauma is permanent. An unimportant and singular exception to this is the regeneration of the fine "fuzz" hairs on the face after dermabrasion.

The portion of the hair within the follicle beneath the surface is the root. The expanded lower part is the bulb that contains the matrix, from which the hair cells are formed. A connective tissue papilla with a capillary loop projects into the base of the bulb. A row of melanocytes is located over the top of the papilla. These furnish melanin for the horny cells coming up from below. Loss of the melanocytic functioning, as in senile graying, has no effect on hair vitality. The matrix is physiologically one of the most intense tissues in the body. Scalp hair grows at an average daily rate of about 0.35 mm., and this is practically all protein (keratin). Hair growth takes place as a holocrine process by the continuous formation of new cells, which move upwards and cornify in a more gradual way than in the epidermis. Interference with cell division in the matrix is immediately reflected in inhibition of hair growth. The rate of cellular reproduction is greater than that of any tissue in the body, with the possible exception of the bone marrow. A highly active tissue of this kind is understandably susceptible to systemic stresses that compromise the general health.

Hair, like nails, grows more rapidly in summer, an expression of an

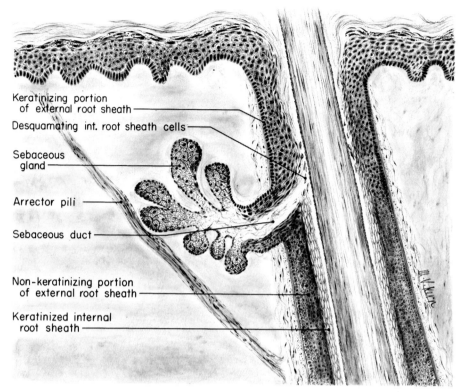

Figure 1–5. Anatomy of the upper region of the follicle

The sebaceous gland is really an appendage of the external root sheath from which it originally develops. The uppermost portion of the external root sheath is a stratified membrane which elaborates keratin in the same manner as the contiguous epidermis. This keratin forms a cylindric tube which closely invests the hair. More deeply within the follicle, approximately in the region of the sebaceous duct, the external root sheath becomes nonstratified and no longer produces keratin. Below this level it is passive. The keratinized internal root sheath cells do not fall apart after their formation below but extend upward as a band, gliding over the surface of the external root sheath. These soft keratin cells desquamate when they reach the level where the external sheath is beginning to produce keratin.

over-all enhancement of cutaneous activity. The hair matrix is a complex tissue that contains a variety of cell types. Its regenerative capacity is astonishing. Forceful manual plucking removes everything but a few torn clusters of matrix cells at the very base. Nonetheless, a perfectly normal hair re-forms from these surviving cells. Within limits, repeated hair plucking does not damage the follicle irreparably, luckily for women who make a lifelong practice of plucking their eyebrows.

A great reduction in hairiness is one of the distinctive features of the human animal. The protection against cold and injury afforded by hair is no longer necessary for civilized man. Over most of the body's surface the hairs are fine and delicate, mere vestiges of their former selves. If hair has lost its biologic significance, its psychologic and cosmetic value has become so much the greater. Too much hair in women and not enough in men have become sensitive issues about which there is extraordinary concern, especially since beauty standards become more exacting and unrealistic with every passing day. As mankind has become more preoccupied with appearance, fictions about hair growth have proliferated.

All over the surface, except the palms, soles and a few other small regions, there are tiny light-colored *vellus* hairs that constitute the "fuzz." These are barely visible, and most people are unaware of their existence. These are the only hairs on the smooth glabrous skin. Even when an individual seems bald, vellus hairs are present. Terminal hairs, by contrast, are long, thick, coarse and darker. They are well developed only in certain regions, such as the scalp, male beard and around the genitalia. From the practical standpoint, terminal hairs are the ones of interest.

Terminal hairs have acquired special characteristics in different regions. This regional diversity is so great that generalizations about hair are not justifiable. For example, scalp and eyelash hairs are quite dissimilar. There are differences in growth rate, anatomic organization and physiologic responsiveness. It is useful to classify hair into six morphologic types: (1) scalp, (2) eyebrow and eyelash, (3) beard, (4) axillary, (5) body and (6) pubic.

Hair may also be divided into two types according to responsiveness to sex hormones. Testosterone controls the postpuberal development of hairs that make up the secondary sex characteristics, that is, the axillary and pubic hair, beard and body hair. On the other hand, scalp hair, eyelashes and hair of the extremities require no hormonal stimulus, although sex hormones may have modifying influences.

The relationship of sex hormones to hair growth has some curious features. It is the male hormone testosterone that governs sex hairs in women as in men. Mustache and facial hair, however, which are hormone-dependent sexual hairs in men, often become prominent in postmenopausal women despite the lack of hormones. Testosterone has completely opposite effects on different types of hairs. It stimulates beard hair for instance, but its presence conditions hair loss in male baldness. Male castrates never become bald. Nor do they have axillary, pubic, beard or body hair. This situation is completely reversed when androgens are given. Eunuchs become "men" in respect to hair. They may lose scalp hair (if there is baldness in the family) and acquire normal hairy characteristics elsewhere. Hormones other than testosterone are generally of little account, either in excess or in deficiency, in affecting hair. It is true that there may be some thinning in hypothyroid myxedema, but this is probably secondary to mucinous infiltration of the skin. The effect of the pituitary is felt indirectly through the production of male hormone by the adrenals and gonads. In rare feminizing disorders of males, excess estrogens may antagonize testosterone to the extent that secondary sex hair regresses.

Hair does not grow indefinitely, as does nail. In every follicle, activity is cyclic — a resting period follows a growth period. The cycles are not synchronized in adjacent follicles. One has a population of independent individual units, each in its own particular phase of the cycle. Some follicles are in infancy while others are in senescence. At the end of the growing phase, the follicle involutes in a remarkable fashion, during which the resting or club hair is formed. This remains passively in the quiescent follicle until it is expelled by the regenerating new hair. A certain number of club hairs are being constantly shed, but since this happens gradually and not all at once, the loss is not perceptible. The situation is analogous to evergreen trees, which, though their limbs are never bare like those of deciduous trees, nonetheless are continuously shedding needles.

Hairs in different regions have different cycles. The main difference is in the length of the growing phase, which determines the final length of

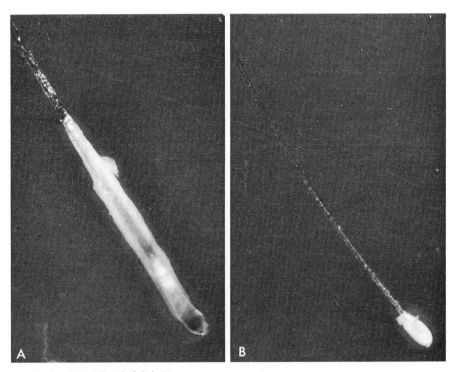

Figure 1–6.   Normal and club hairs

Plucking the hair will show whether it is growing or resting (provided it does not break off).

A. A growing hair. The hair root is surrounded by an extensive translucent sheath and the proximal tip is deeply pigmented. The hair itself may be seen within the sheath.

B. A resting or club hair. All that is seen is a bulbous, nonpigmented tip. There is no sheath save for an inconspicuous one limited to the very tip of the hair. Club hairs are also likely to be somewhat lighter and thinner, because pigment production and keratin synthesis diminish when the hair nears the end of the growing phase.

the hair. Short hairs obviously come from follicles with brief growing phases. It is roughly estimated that scalp hair grows for from 2 to 6 years. Actually, the hairs of certain persons may grow for 25 years. This must be true, else in times past it would have been impossible for some women to grow hair down to their knees, assuming an average daily growth rate of 0.35 mm. Resting hairs make up about 5 to 15 per cent of the terminal scalp hairs. Since the great majority of the approximately 100,000 hairs on the human scalp are growing at any given time, the resting period must be short, perhaps a matter of a few months. The normal rate of scalp hair loss is in the range of 20 to 100 hairs daily. Most of the inconspicuous vellus hairs of the body will be found to be in the resting phase.

On the trunk, eyebrows and extremities, the growing period usually does not exceed six months, hence the hairs are not very long. These hairs rest for about the same length of time as they grow. Appreciation of the cyclical habit of hair growth has practical applications. Hair infection by the ringworm fungus *Microsporum audouini* is automatically cured when hairs enter the resting phase. It is easy to understand, then, why infections of the eyelashes and eyelids terminate spontaneously in a couple of months; such hairs are in a growing phase only for this long. In the scalp, however, the infection may last for years if treatment with griseofulvin is not instituted.

A variety of systemic stresses, especially acute febrile diseases, may interfere with hair growth and structure. It is scalp hair that is particularly vulnerable. A shortening of the life cycle, with premature formation of resting hairs, is one striking result. This may never become clinically apparent if gradual and limited, but if a majority of hairs are suddenly brought into a synchronous resting phase, their loss shortly thereafter will be accompanied by signs of thinning and even baldness. This effect is generally temporary, since loss of normal resting hairs is regularly followed by regeneration of new hairs. More chronic stresses, by shortening the life cycles, cause more rapid turnover in the hair crop. More hairs are being lost and regenerated. As long as the birth rate of hairs equals the death rate, there may be thinning but not real baldness. It becomes important, therefore, to be able to recognize a club hair. In male baldness and in scarring diseases, the follicle shrivels and the hairs wither away, so that regeneration is impossible.

There are a number of situations in which there is temporary partial baldness owing to the loss of an unusual number of resting hairs. This happens physiologically in infants within the first few months after birth. Postpartum hair loss is a very common phenomenon in mothers. The stress of the delivery and the physiologic drains of pregnancy are reflected in a goodly percentage of cases in the formation of a large number of club hairs. This premature shortening of the cycles may happen suddenly or over a period of months. Hair loss is very noticeable in the former case but is merely an accentuation of a physiologic process. It abates spontaneously. Chronic emotional stress, debilitating disease of diverse origin and, occasionally, profound malnutrition are responsible for similar phenomena.

The peculiar susceptibility of scalp hair is evident in other ways. Moderate doses of thallium acetate will cause depilation of scalp hair but not other types of hair. Survivors of the atom bombings in Japan lost only their scalp hair (in the absence of scarring). The fact that scalp hair grows faster than other types may help to account for its sensitivity. Eyebrow hairs grow at half this rate. It takes three to four months for scalp hair to be restored after plucking but only a month or so for short-cycle, slow-growing hair like the eyebrow.

The scalp hair, like the nails, tends to reflect systemic illness and health-weakening stresses, again in no specific manner. The body has more important functions to perform at such times. Hair growth may slow down; the hairs may become thinner, more fragile, split and, in other ways, poor in appearance.

Misconceptions about hair growth are legion. This simply reflects the tremendous psychologic significance of hair. One source of error among serious students has been unwarranted applications of results of animal research. The skin and hair of common laboratory animals, such as the mouse, rabbit and rat, have unique properties. Procedures or drugs that

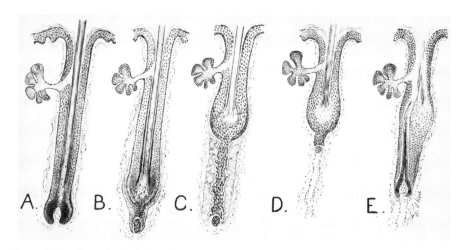

Figure 1–7.   Stages in the hair cycle

A. Growing hair.

B. Presumptive club. The matrix is involuted and no longer producing differentiated keratinized cells. The papilla is becoming free.

C. Emergent club. The matrix cells have formed a column which has pushed the club outwards.

D. Mature club. The epithelial column has retracted by disorganization of most of its cells. The papilla has moved up proportionately as the column has shortened. The papilla persists through the entire cycle. The hair itself is inserted into a sac of undifferentiated epithelial cells. Some of these are removed when the hair is plucked, forming a thin sheath around the base of the hair.

E. New hair formation.

will correct graying in animals or stimulate new hair growth, matters of exceeding concern to many humans, have not proved useful in clinical medicine. Among widely believed myths are the following: shaving promotes the growth of dark, coarse hairs; singeing and cutting the hair weaken it; hair can turn gray overnight; hair "grows after death"; and so forth.

It should be realized that the hair shaft is a dead, inert structure. No force, chemical or physical, that is confined exactly to this structure can possibly alter the hair-forming organ, which is situated well under the scalp's surface and is, therefore, not easily harmed. As for massage, combing, brushing, oiling and a thousand other practices thought to improve hair growth — none has established value. These activities are cosmetically satisfying but do not improve upon nature's capacity to produce healthy hair. Cleanliness is the only essential in maintaining scalp health. Everything else is for appearance.

The importance of vitamins on hair growth has been much exaggerated. No single vitamin has a pronounced influence. Nor is hair loss a particularly striking result of vitamin deficiency. It is only in advanced malnutrition, particularly with prolonged protein privation, that fragility or loss of hair becomes evident.

NAILS

The nail plate is a hard *keratin* structure. Its horny cells are cemented together tightly and do not separate, as do stratum corneum cells. Nails can, thus, extend indefinitely unless cut or broken. Nails more than a foot long, once a custom in some countries, were an indubitable sign of wealth. At an average growth rate of about 0.1 mm. a day, it takes a fingernail about 3.5 months to be replaced if it is lost. Like hair, nails grow more rapidly in the summer.

Toenails grow much more slowly than fingernails, especially in older persons. A variety of nonspecific nail changes occur in response to systemic stresses. By and large these changes are not characteristic enough to suggest a specific diagnosis. In prolonged fevers, drug reactions, chemical toxemias and advanced malnutrition, the nail may be shed altogether, or there may be various degress of thinning, thickening, splitting, ridging and furrowing. Even emotional stresses may be reflected in abnormal nails. Nails are not vital to life; in times of stress the body reserves are used for other purposes and the nails are "allowed" to suffer. To some extent the nail reflects the general state of body health, although this relationship is irregular and the changes not distinctive. The nails of malnourished children have been found to grow more slowly. Contrary to popular opinion vitamin deficiencies and dietary irregularities do not quickly manifest themselves in nail abnormalities. Unhappily, fragile, brittle, thinned or split nails occur quite frequently in the absence of any discernible abuse. The nails, along with the skin, show deterioration with aging.

Diseases serious enough to affect the nails often involve the hair, again in the same nonspecific manner, such as slowing of growth, thinning, breaking and shedding. These two hard keratin structures form a clinicopathologic couplet. There are singular instances in which the student of rare signs can astonish his colleagues with an unusual diagnosis derived solely from inspection of the nails. For instance, in the nephrotic syndrome, when the serum albumin falls below 2.2 gm. per 100 ml., two transverse white bands may form at the base of the nails. Transverse white bands may signify arsenical poisoning to the nail sleuth. Few such opportunities are presented!

Attention is called to the fact that this section deals mainly with fingernails, not toenails. The latter are somewhat different anatomically and their clinical significance is minor. Toenails have little useful function in a shoe-wearing civilization.

Nails are quick to reflect local stresses. Persistent trauma in some occupations may lead to great thickening. Nail biting may almost double

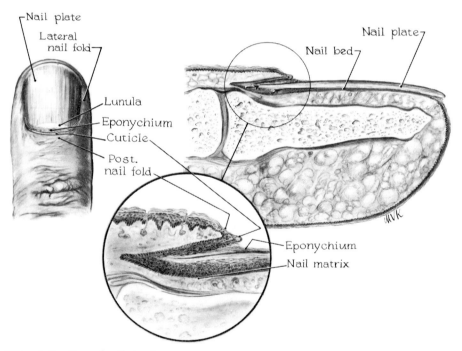

Figure 1–8.   Normal nail structure

The angle of insertion of the nail into the skin is very small, so that the epithelial invagination in which it is born (its follicle) is practically parallel to the skin's surface. The nail grows in the long axis of its "follicle" as does a hair. The epithelium at the base of the invagination is the generative zone, or matrix, and may be seen to be continuous with the nail bed anteriorly and with the posterior nail fold above and posteriorly. The matrix is not a highly specialized structure. Note how closely it is apposed to bone.

the rate of growth. Dermatitis of the distal digit secondarily compromises nail growth and form. Changes in the plate are, of course, permanent "scars," a result of prior injury to the nail-forming organ. These "scars" are eliminated when the nail grows out.

The nail plate is colorless and without melanin pigment. The varying colors from pink to white are determined by the way incident light is reflected from the underlying structures. The free edge of the nail is grayish white, owing to free air beneath it. Accordingly, whenever the nail separates from its bed in pathologic conditions, it becomes whitish. The pink color of the major portion of the plate reflects the rich vascular plexus in the nail bed. Pressure blanches the nail by forcing blood out of the capillaries. The lunula is a semilunar white region at the base of the plate, generally found in the thumbnail of all persons and to a variable and progressively lesser degree in more lateral fingers. It corresponds to an underlying cushion of epithelial cells from which the nail springs, the nail matrix. Keratinizing cells in this area reflect white light. The rest of the matrix is hidden beneath the posterior nail fold. Where there is no lunula, the matrix extends under the nail fold for 0.5 to 1.0 cm. Whenever cellular keratinization is incomplete and nuclei persist, white spots or streaks, called leukonychia, are the result. These are exceedingly common, coming and going in a will-of-the-wisp fashion; they have no significance other than being temporary imperfections.

The nail bed is the tissue under that portion of the plate that appears pink. Its epithelial lining is passive and inert in the sense that it forms no keratin and does not contribute to the plate at all. The plate simply glides over the nail bed, receiving no substance or sustenance as it moves. The union between the plate and the epithelium of the bed, however, is of the firmest possible sort, so much so that during avulsion of the nail, the line of separation is the junction of the epithelium with the corium, not the plate and the epithelium. In short, the whole epithelium is ripped away. Because of this extraordinary adhesion, the plate and the epithelium move outward together at the same rate, the latter possibly being dragged along by the former. This is the reason why a hematoma that forms subungually does not remain in place but gradually moves outward with the growth of the nail, a form of physiologic debridement. India ink placed beneath the nail into the bed similarly migrates outwards and is expelled at the distal border.

The nail bed epithelium keratinizes distally, producing a yellowish discolored surface band just proximal to where the nail separates from the bed. Under pathologic conditions the nail bed abandons its passive state and is converted into a stratified keratinizing membrane. Horny masses pile up under the plate with resultant thickening deformation and, sometimes, separation of the plate from its bed. Inflammatory lesions of the nail bed invariably cause subungual accumulations of horny debris, a quite characteristic change in certain disorders, such as psoriasis and ringworm infection.

Fine longitudinal ridges are seen to a variable degree in the normal

trogens, for instance, darken the nipples, but melanocytes elsewhere are not activated. Thus the melanocytes may be classified into morphologic and physiologic varieties.

The *skin of darkly pigmented races* does not contain *more* melanocytes. They are simply larger and work harder. It is not number but function that is decisive. In the ordinary pigmented freckle, melanocytes are actually fewer than in the surrounding skin. When there is no pigmentation at all, as

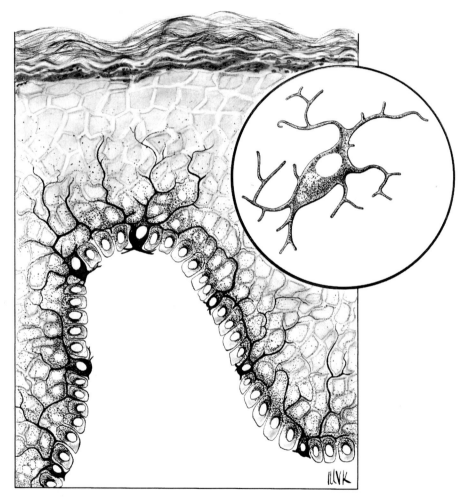

Figure 1–9. Melanocytes in epidermis

The melanin-forming cells are situated among the basal cells. They have long branching cell processes or tubes through which the pigment granules are carried to be "injected" into the remaining nonmelanin-forming cells of the epidermis. The melanin often forms a supranuclear cap of pigment granules in the basal cells. The inset shows a single melanocyte with its elaborate branches.

in the genetic condition of albinism or in acquired vitiligo, melanocytes are present in the usual numbers but the synthesis of melanin is blocked. The factories are there but are not in operation. There are no primary diseases characterized solely by absence of melanocytes.

The melanin made by melanocytes does not always end up in epidermal cells. In various pathologic states, especially if there is much inflammation, some may escape into the dermis where it is ingested by phagocytic cells. These cells "mop up" free melanin just as they would carbon particles and are called melanophages or melanophores. In metastatic malignant melanoma, the whole skin may darken, owing to tremendous deposition of melanin granules within melanophages and in the corium.

Melanin formation is an enzymic process, the details of which are fairly well understood. The biochemical requisites are: (1) the amino acid tyrosine, (2) a copper-containing enzyme, tyrosinase, and (3) molecular oxygen. Tyrosinase oxidizes tyrosine to dihydroxyphenylalanine (dopa). Dopa undergoes further transformation to dopaquinone and thence through a complex series of metabolic steps involving indoles, finally ending in melanin. When a fresh sheet of epidermis is incubated in tyrosine, new melanin is formed in the melanocytes, and the cells look darker. When there is a clinical deficiency of tyrosine, as in phenylketonuria, the skin stays light. Conversely, the hyperpigmentation seen in liver disease may be due to excessive accumulation of tyrosine in the blood. The first awareness that only certain epidermal cells make melanin came through the discovery that only melanocytes became darker when section of skin were immersed in dopa. This was attributed to dopa-oxidase (now known to be tyrosinase), present only in melanin-synthesizing cells. The dopa reaction is still the easiest way to identify melanocytes physiologically. Dopa, however, can be oxidized by nonspecific oxidases present universally in tissues, and proper care must be exerted. Even leukocytes are dopa-positive. After irradiation with ultraviolet light or x-rays, the tyrosinase system is activated, and epidermis incubated in dopa or tyrosine gets darker. It is thought that there is some inhibiting substance which holds tyrosinase in check, perhaps a sulfhydryl-containing compound that binds the copper of the enzyme. A water-soluble sulfhydrl substance that inhibits the tyrosinase system in vitro has been extracted from skin. Evidently, there is less of it in Negro skin and so tyrosinase is more free to act. Agencies that inactivate sulfhydryl groups promote tanning and include arsenic, x-rays and inflammation.

Substances that inhibit the tyrosinase reaction have potential applicability as *depigmenting agents*. The best known of these, monobenzyl ether of hydroquinone, an antioxidant used in the rubber industry, formerly caused occupational depigmentation. This substance is used topically for therapeutic depigmentation of unsightly hyperpigmentation. The response is slow, requiring application over weeks and months, probably because the impermeability of skin limits the amount reaching the melanocytes in the basal layer. Moreover the compound frequently produces sensitization reactions. Parenteral administration of a number of hyroquinones depigments animal skin.

Curiously, melanin becomes colorless when further oxidized. This is the basis of bleaching with hydrogen peroxide. Strong sunlight has this effect to a lesser extent, and dark hair often becomes light or develops reddish tints in the summer. The chemical intermediates before melanin are also colorless but become pigmented upon oxidation. Even the skin of a cadaver will "tan" slightly after heat or irradiation because of this conversion (Meirowsky phenomenon).

The controlling forces of melanin synthesis are complex, partly local and partly systemic. Hormonal and neurogenic agencies are among the latter. As regards susceptibility of melanocytes to purely local happenings, inflammation, no matter how produced (chemical, physical, thermal, infectious), is the commonest and most important source of increased melanogenesis. Pigmentation is one of the most certain signs of previous dermatitis and is characteristic of the healing phase. On the other hand, severely inflammatory processes may utterly destroy or at least batter melanocytes so that no pigment can be formed until new melanocytes migrate in or the remaining ones can recover. Occasionally, even a mild disorder such as tinea versicolor is associated with depigmentation; in these instances, the melanocytes are intact but there is enzymic interference. Melanocytes function independently of keratinocytes. X-rays may cause complete and permanent depigmentation of animal hair without interfering with its growth.

Hormones play a prominent general role in influencing melanogenesis in health and disease. The most specific and important of these is produced by the intermediate (possibly the anterior) lobe of the pituitary through the melanocyte-stimulating hormone, generally abbreviated MSH. With large doses of MSH a diffuse pigmentation, more intense on exposed areas, may become apparent in 24 hours. Over a period of weeks, a white person's skin may beome as dark as a black's. Urinary excretion of MSH is the same in blacks, whites and albinos, indicating that the pigmentary differences are due to the intrinsic capacity of the target cells to respond to the hormonal stimulus. The immediate darkening of isolated frog skin in MSH solutions provides a sensitive assay for its presence. MSH is chemically similar to ACTH. Indeed, ACTH will cause some hyperpigmentation, possibly because it is contaminated with MSH. As expected, skin lightens after hypophysectomy, and there is no MSH in the urine. This is also evident in states of hypopituitarism. Cortisone and its analogues inhibit the secretion of MSH; therefore, in Addison's disease and after adrenalectomy, increased MSH from the pituitary causes diffuse darkening of the skin. Administration of corticosteroids to such patients lightens the skin. In this way a controlling effect is exerted by the pituitary adrenal axis.

Increased pigmentation is an occasional phenomenon in patients with a variety of central nervous system disorders, such as encephalitis and brain tumors. This also happens in psychotic states. Presumably these diverse processes cause the pituitary to secrete larger amounts of MSH or possibly ACTH. It is an ancient observation that anxiety may cause darkening under the eyes, perhaps by this same mechanism. MSH is also increased in pregnancy.

Other hormones play a subsidiary role in pigmentation. Estrogens darken the nipples, even when applied topically. Eunuchs do not tan properly after sunlight exposure. The administration of testosterone corrects this. It is well to mention that skin color is not solely a reflection of melanin. Blood pigments and oxidized and reduced hemoglobin also contribute to normal skin color. A poor vascular supply, as in hypogonadal states, makes the skin appear lighter. The more normal color after sex hormone therapy is largely due to improved vasculature. Epinephrine antagonizes the effect of MSH on the target cell, at least in isolated frog skin.

A possible direct neurogenic control of pigmentation is a fascinating hypothesis. Melanocytes have been likened to nerve cells because their dendrites look like axons; moreover they originate from the neural crest. Interruption of the sympathetics in fish leads to a pronounced darkening of the denervated segment. An indirect piece of evidence in man is the remarkable occurrence of dark café au lait spots in von Recklinghausen's neurofibromatosis.

Changes in melanin pigmentation are a conspicuous feature of many dermatologic disorders, and their observation is, thus, an important element in dermatologic diagnosis. It should be remembered that pigmentary changes are not always due to melanin; intrinsic pigments such as bilirubin and hemosiderin, and extrinsic pigments, such as silver and bismuth, may discolor skin.

SKIN PERMEABILITY

It is the *impermeability* of normal skin that is one of its chief protective devices. This generalization, however, is not absolute. Certain classes of substances go through skin more readily than others. The advantage of applying medicaments directly to diseased skin is counteracted by the skin's resistance to their penetration. In many diseases, though the skin lesions seem superficial and available for influence by topical agents, it is very difficult to achieve adequate concentrations of the therapeutic agents within the lesions.

Substances may enter the skin by passing directly through the epidermis, the transepidermal route, or via the orifices of the follicles. If the epidermis could not be bypassed through these follicular "holes," the skin would be even less permeable than it is. It is necessary to emphasize that very sensitive techniques, such as radioautography, will almost always show some degree of penetrability for any substance. Our discussion is concerned with permeability at the clinical or biologic level of significance.

To enter transepidermally, a substance must first get through the horny layer. This structure is not so porous as formerly thought. The overlapping layers of imbricated cells are not easily penetrated. Even water does not leak through quickly, else a purely intracorneal blister, as in sweat retention vesicles, would be impossible. The resistance of ringworm infections, characteristically limited to the stratum corneum, to topical antifungal medication is another proof of the chemical insulation afforded by the horny layer. The thick, dense, horny later of the palms and soles is essentially impenetrable. This is why, for instance, the palms are often exempt from allergic contact dermatitis.

The *barrier to epidermal penetration* is said to be located directly under-

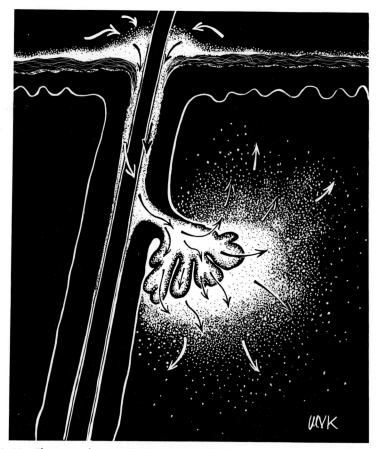

Figure 1–10.   The route of penetration into normal skin

Many substances capable of penetrating the skin gain entrance through follicular orifices and pass through the sebaceous gland, thus bypassing the epidermal barrier. Other substances, however, damage and pass directly through the epidermal barrier into the connective tissue, blood vessels, and lymphatics within the dermis.

neath the stratum corneum in the transitional zone. Whatever the true case, it is certainly the outermost, mostly nonviable portion of the epidermis which serves this function. The absence of a true stratum corneum and a transitional zone in the mucous membranes of the mouth enables ready penetration. Many drugs are put up in a form suitable for transmucosal absorption in the mouth. As a simple example, the mouth and the cornea, but not the skin, can be easily anesthetized by topical application of various agents.

Disruption of the anatomic barrier of the outer epidermis decreases the skin's impermeability greatly. It then becomes leaky and porous. Minor trauma, such as stripping a few times with cellophane tape or "dry shaving" with a sharp blade, can weaken the barrier. Inflammation greatly increases absorption of topically applied substances. Skin without an epidermis, as in erosions or ulcers is freely permeable. The more extensive the damage, the more permeable the skin becomes. Boric acid compresses on an extensive dermatits may cause death through boron poisoning, although absorption of boric acid through intact skin is negligble.

By entering the follicular orifices, substances can bypass the epidermal barrier altogether. If miscible or soluble in fat, they can seep down into the sebaceous duct and pass through the sebaceous gland, fanning out from there into the dermis. *The pilosebaceous route is the chief means of transit through the skin.* Penetration is, therefore, best in densely hairy areas. Conversely, absence of follicles in atrophic or senile skin lowers permeability.

Regional differences in permeability are considerable, owing to differences in thickness of the epidermis and the number and size of follicles. The sweat ducts evidently do not serve as a route of ingress. A striking way to demonstrate follicular absorption is to place 5 per cent aqueous solutions of histamine or norepinephrine on the hairy forearm. Little perifollicular wheals and blanched areas (with piloerection) form, respectively. Washing the skin first with soap and water, or prior defatting with ether or chloroform, somewhat enhances penetrability of the above agents from aqueous solution. Although this is possibly due to removal of surface fats, enabling the water solution to wet the follicle orifice, the surface lipids usually play an insignificant role in preventing absorption. The first prerequisite for achieving maximal absorption is to enable the substance to enter the follicle. Rubbing will do this to some extent by forcing the agent into the orifices. Merely dabbing a medicament onto the skin is inadeaquate. It should be firmly rubbed on. Occlusion of the site under an impermeable dressing also facilitates penetration. Ointments are often preferred as vehicles because they can be pressed into the follicles, are not easily removed and stick to the surface for a long time. It should always be remembered that damaging the epidermis increases permeability, whether this is done mechanically by rubbing and scratching or chemically by using irritating vehicles or substances. Simple hyperemia does not enhance the skin's penetrability.

Three main factors are involved in the formal analysis of skin permeability:

1. The *structural organization* of the skin (thickness, presence of appendages, anatomical integrity, etc.). This has been discussed above.

2. The *vehicle or base*, a topic with endless possiblities but limited accomplishment.

3. The *substance itself*.

Dermatologists have understandably been greatly preoccupied with vehicles, pinning high hopes on developing formulations that would "solve" the problem of getting things into the skin. This ambition has not been realized except by occlusion with a polyethylene film. The chief progress has been in preparing pharmaceutically elegant bases that are acceptable to the patient. Messy, disagreeable, uncosmetic formulations are a thing of the past. Out of this effort has come a hard awareness of the physiologic facts of skin penetrability, though misconceptions are still legion, and vendors of vehicles still lure the gullible with promises of increased efficacy. In vitro studies have little or no correlation with in vivo performance.

The subject of skin penetration is full of ambiguities and contradictions owing to oversimplification that fail to take into account the numerous variables that are operative. Generalizations are helpful for didactic purposes, but exceptions are numerous. The firm rules are so few that one has to fall back on experience and the empirical legacies left by generations of skilled dermatologic therapists.

It should be clearly understood that vehicles do not and cannot carry substances through the skin directly. If the skin is basically impermeable to a given substance, no vehicle will transport it through (unless it is damaging). The penetrabilities of the vehicle and its incorporated substance are independent variables. A given substance, however, will penetrate better from certain vehicles than others. For instance, salicylic acid penetrates better from lanolin than from petrolatum, although both are immiscible in water, and this result could not have been predicted. Greater or lesser penetration from vehicles is largely a matter of complex physical factors, most of them poorly defined, such as rate of release, solubility, capacity to emulsify with skin oils and water, adhesiveness and viscosity. The primary role of the vehicle is to bring the substance into optimum anatomic contact with the skin, that is, to deliver it to the "gates" and to release it. If it succeeds in getting through, it will be because the gates are open; the skin, in short, is permeable. There is no absolute law that can be laid down for selecting a vehicle; the only valid generalization is the one stating that each substance is a law unto itself. The optimum vehicle must be determined empirically for each substance, an obviously impractical task. There is no *universally superior*, all-purpose vehicle. Furthermore, to maintain clinical perspective one should never lose sight of the relative impermeability of the skin; the amount that gets through in any case is small. For these reasons the vehicle does not have the importance usually ascribed to it. Certain empirical rules dealing with the skin's tolerance and patient acceptability are more important guides than elegant theoretical considerations. Finally, it is well to admit the possibility that a topical agent may be effective, even though its penetrability is minimal. By not passing through too quickly, it may be concentrated in the very area where it will do the most good.

Substances vary greatly in their penetrability. Although strict generalizations are impossible, it is useful to make a classification of chemical groups that will tell something about the likelihood of penetration. The first is that fat-soluble substances tend to go through skin. Some degree of water solubility is also favorable. Substances that are completely insoluble in water and lipids do not penetrate. The penetrability of any particular agent in this lipoid-water soluble class, however, is not predictable beforehand from an inspection of its solubility characteristics; it does not follow that hight lipoid solubility is invariably associated with high penetrability. Again, empirical considerations are sovereign; other variables interfere with generalizations. For instance, the original substance, say a mercuric salt, may form a compound of greater solubility by combining with the fatty acids of sebum. In its transformed state it may get in more easily. By various interactions with substances on the surface, an originally lipoid-insoluble agent may be converted into one with more favorable chemical solubility for penetration. Vehicles, too, may enter into such reactions. As a rule, neither proteins nor carbohydrates enter skin, possibly because of large molecular size and lipid insolubility. That trace amounts can go through does not negate the rule. The Vollmer patch test causes a reaction in tuberculin-sensitive persons precisely because tiny amounts of tuberculoprotein can excite an allergic response in the highly sensitive. Similarly, putting egg white on the normal skin may cause an attack of asthma in the exquisitely sensitive patient.

A brief résumé of penetrability according to chemical class follows:

WATER.   Water is lost transepidermally as insensible perspiration. This is a one-way street. Water does not enter the skin appreciably from the outside.

ELECTROLYTES.   Electrolytes cannot pass through the skin appreciably. This is partly due to electrical properties of skin that counteract the passage of charged ions. The epidermis behaves as a negatively charged membrane. Accordingly, negatively charged anions are repelled, and ionized salts are not easily admitted. A practical illustration of this is the fact that the sodium salt of salicylic acid will not penetrate the skin from any base whereas salicylic acid does so. The rule is that the free base, not the salt, should be used when penetration is desired.

An electrical force may be used to help propel electrolytes into skin, but the substance must first have some degree of penetrability of its own. Iontophoresis, as this process is called, is a form of electrophoresis in which charged particles migrate in an electric field. Iontophoresis merely accelerates the rate of entry with an electric "push"; it will not make a substance go through if the skin is completely impermeable to this compound.

GASES.   All true gases except carbon monoxide pass directly through skin. This is the only class of substances to which the skin is freely permeable. If a tourniquet is placed around the arm until it becomes cyanotic, a normal pink color may redevelop if the occluded limb is placed in an atmosphere of oxygen.

LIPIDS.   A variety of different lipids may be absorbed through the skin. Fat-soluble vitamins and steroid hormones are notable examples. Vitamins A and D penetrate quite readily. Indeed, vitamin D is made on the skin's surface by the action of sunlight on its precursor; its absorption is a physiologic phenomenon. This does not mean that the topical application of these vitamins is good for skin, normal or diseased. Estrogens are sufficiently absorbed to cause menstrual irregularities, breast enlargement and hyperpigmentation. Topical application of testosterone may cause hair to grow in the axillae of eunuchs.

There are no practical indications for giving vitamins and hormones via the skin route except for rare instances in which a purely local effect might be desired.

Lipid-soluble alkaloid bases such as strychnine, nicotine and opium are readily absorbed. Not so their salts. Animals die when rubbed with strychnine base ointment but are unharmed by strychnine sulfate.

THE GLANDS OF THE SKIN

The Sebaceous Gland

Specialization of skin function is further reflected by three different glandular appendages: the sebaceous gland, the apocrine gland and the eccrine sweat gland. These are all of epidermal origin and may be viewed as specialized cellular invaginations. The sebaceous gland is a holocrine unit that continuously forms a complex lipoidal mixture known as sebum. The cells that form the gland all differentiate into fatty materials, which on dissolution of the cell membranes flow out over the skin surface. Chemically, this sebum may be characterized as composed of free fatty acids, esterified fatty acids and unsaponifiable compounds such as cholesterol, squalene and other hydrocarbons. It also contains some pro-vitamin D, 7-dehydrocholesterol. By the action of ultraviolet light this is converted into vitamin D and reabsorbed.

The sebaceous glands are not grossly visible except in an aberrant localization in the oral mucous membranes. Here they appear as clusters of grouped yellowish masses, a characteristic of Fordyce's disease. Local overgrowths of the sebaceous gland (senile sebaceous adenomas) are commonly seen on the aging skin of the face. Sebaceous glands normally are found only in association with hair follicles. Paradoxically, there is often an inverse relationship between the size of the gland and that of the hair. Thus, fine lanugo hairs of the face may be associated with very large

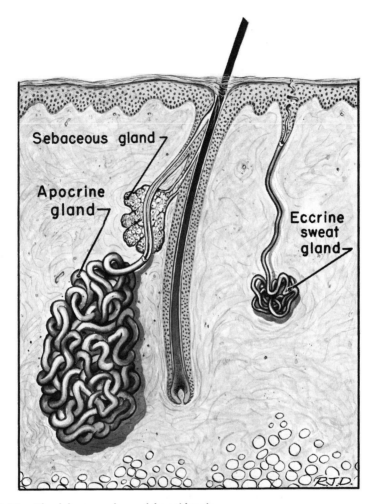

Figure 1–11. Glandular appendages of the epidermis

Schematic cross-sectional drawing of the glandular appendages of the epidermis. Note that the apocrine gland and sebaceous gland have a common final excretory pathway. See Figure 1–12 for the areas in which the apocrine gland is found.

sebaceous glands. The gland is actually an outpouching of the follicular wall and ordinarily rests just above the arrector pili muscle. It is covered not with any specialized sheath but with just a simple connective tissue capsule. Although it is richly supplied with blood vessels, no nerve supply is demonstrable. The gland is multilobulated and possesses no true excretory duct other than the passage up the hair follicle.

The distribution of the sebaceous glands is of striking clinical significance. On the face, scalp and scrotum one finds them in greatest abundance. Excessive production of sebum is called seborrhea, and this occurs where the glands are normally found in large numbers. Lesser numbers of sebaceous glands are found on the upper trunk and there is a progressive diminution in density on the extremities. On the dorsum of the hands and feet very few glands are present. Oil glands are entirely absent on the palms and soles. These areas depend largely on passively transferred sebum and on inherent lipids for lubrication. In considering the mechanism of lubrication of the normal skin, a second line of defense is to be found in the epidermis itself, which forms lipids, although to a lesser extent. Thus, the desquamating keratinocyte, although predominantly keratin, also contains lipids that are found in the surface film.

Area differences in sebum formation are striking, but no less so are age and individual variations in this respect. The oily skin of puberty is striking, as is the dry skin surface of old age. The skin of persons in the tropics is commonly oily, whereas the skin of the northern inhabitants is known for its tendency to dry out and to develop "winter itch." Finally, sebaceous activity is greater in the male than in the female, as a rule.

The emergence of sebum on the skin surface is ordinarily a constant, imperceptible process, in marked contrast to the intermittent flow of either apocrine or eccrine sweat. For this reason, study of the physiology of sebum formation has been difficult. Actually, however, some simple tests are of help in interpreting the functioning of the sebaceous gland. It is possible to assay the rate of sebum delivery simply by wiping off the free surface oil with soft absorbent paper; after thirty minutes, brief application of a clean glass microscope slide will provide a print of the degree of oiliness. Indeed, simple inspection of oily skin will disclose numerous sparkling droplets of a clear fluid, which is actually sebum but almost invariably passes for eccrine sweat. Distinction between sebum and sweat rests on the fact that sweat will evaporate rapidly from the glass slide.

Sebum formation and secretion is a simple growth process. There is no direct neural influence. Drugs are not known to affect the secretory rate. In warm environments sebum formation is accelerated, presumably due to the elevated skin temperature. Sebum formation and secretion are not affected by simple physical factors, such as the presence of ointment on the skin. The gland is refractory to all but massive doses of x-ray. Permanent destruction of the sebaceous gland is achieved only with the administration of dosages well beyond the safe therapeutic range. The fact that the sebaceous glands undergo such a marked hypertrophy at puberty clearly indicates hormonal control of them. Large doses of androgens in animals cause hypertrophy of the glands, and estrogens cause involution. Recent studies suggest that a pituitary hormone is responsible, but as yet there is no safe method of producing diminution of sebum production clinically.

The Apocrine Gland

The apocrine gland is a vestigial skin appendage of no known physiologic significance. Its importance in dermatology stems from the fact that it

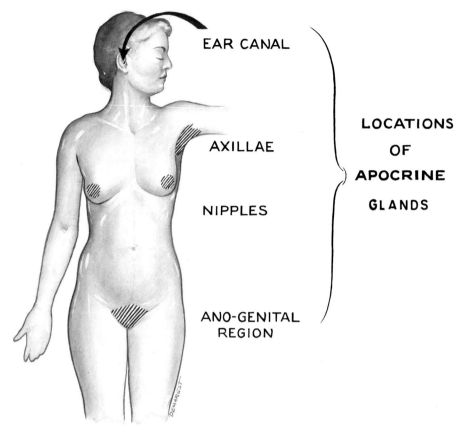

EAR CANAL

AXILLAE

NIPPLES

ANO-GENITAL
REGION

LOCATIONS

OF

APOCRINE

GLANDS

Figure 1–12.   Distribution of apocrine glands

In man the apocrine glands are normally found only in certain areas. The apocrine glands in the ear canal form ear wax. In addition to the sites shown above, apocrine glands are found in a vestigial form in the eyelids (glands of Moll).

may be responsible for certain body odors and that it is the site of certain disease states. Though it is commonly designated as a "sweat" gland, its secretion is entirely different from that of the eccrine gland.

Basically, the apocrine gland is the specialized gland of the axilla. It is here that the gland is found in its greatest size and density. It is not widely distributed, as are the sebaceous and eccrine glands. Indeed, its restricted localization is of aid in indicating that certain diseases limited to these same areas are of apocrine origin. The typical sites for apocrine glands are the axillae, the areolae of the nipples and the periumbilical, perianal and genital regions. Elsewhere the glands are ectopic and unusual. Two specialized exceptions are to be noted. Atrophic apocrine glands are to be found in the eyelid, the glands of Moll. The most common pathologic change in these is cystic, due to poral blockage. The second area of special apocrine glands is the ear canal. Here the glands secrete a portion of what is seen as ear wax. Parenthetically, it may be stated that, from the evolutionary standpoint, the apocrine gland reaches its ultimate functional status as the mammary gland.

As a rule, the apocrine gland, like the sebaceous gland, is attached to the hair follicle. The gland is a simple, coiled, tubular gland. It is considerably larger than the sebaceous or eccrine gland. There is a long duct leading down from the hair follicle to the coil of secretory tubules. These tubules are surrounded by a thin sheath of contractile tissue known as myoepithelium. This myoepithelium, in turn, is supplied by a fine network of adrenergic nerves.

Apocrine secretion is a milkish white fluid that appears on the skin in very minute quantities. It appears at the instant of emotional stress, such as fear or anger. Individuals vary greatly in their capacity for apocrine sweating but in none is the secretion of any volume. Indeed, apocrine sweating is completely masked by concomitant eccrine sweating. It is of no significance to the normal individual other than that numerous surface bacteria feed upon the fats of apocrine sweat, producing variably pungent odors. Apocrine secretion is sterile and odorless as it comes on the skin surface. It is the later, secondary bacterial changes that account for the distinctive odor. In the absence of apocrine sweating, as in prepuberty or in senescence, the axilla is odorless.

Functionally, the apocrine gland is unique. Unlike the eccrine and sebaceous glands (and the ear canal gland), it does not function at all in the child. Only at puberty does it awaken in response to the same sex hormonal influences that cause development of the hair of the axilla. It is, thus, a sex characteristic.

The secretory cells function slowly and continuously, forming secretion just as in the case of milk. This remains in the gland lumen, to be expelled by myoepithelial contraction at times of stress. The myoepithelial sheath contracts in response to adrenergic impulses or to circulating smooth muscle stimulants such as epinephrine or oxytocin (Pitocin). Once an individual gland has been disengorged of its tiny droplet, further stress or stimulation of that gland is ineffective until more secretion has accumulated.

Recent studies, with great potential for the clinical treatment of acne, have shown that the oral administration of 13-cis-retinoic acid produces significant reduction of sebum secretion.*

The Eccrine Sweat Gland

In contrast to the unobtrusive and relatively inapparent activity of the sebaceous and apocrine glands, the functioning of the eccrine gland is most

---

*Strauss, N. S., Peck, C. L., Olsen, T. G., Downing, D. T., and Windhorst, D. B.: Alteration of skin lipid composition by oral 13-cis-retinoic acid: Comparison of pretreatment and treatment values. J. Invest. Dermatol. 70:223, 1978.

obvious. It produces a product that is at once felt and seen and that is essential to thermoregulation. These glands have a far more uniform and generalized distribution pattern than other appendages, though certain areas are more richly endowed, e.g., the forehead, the palms and the soles. All told, several million eccrine sweat units are ready for instant functioning in response to a heat stimulus.

The gland itself is composed of a duct opening in a free invisible pore and a secretory coil deep in the corium. Only a vestigial myoepithelium enwraps the coil, and this has no proven function. Numerous cholinergic nerves supply the secretory portion of the gland. Master control of all of the eccrine glands is achieved through the heat regulatory center of the hypothalamus. This, in turn, activates the sympathetic fibers, which, paradoxi-

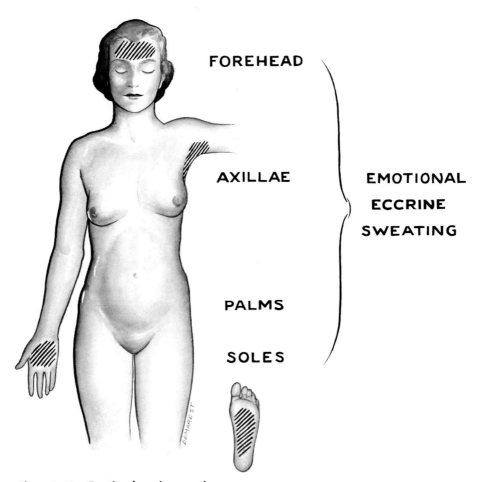

Figure 1–13. Emotional eccrine sweating

Eccrine sweating induced by emotional stimuli appears characteristically in certain areas, as illustrated above. Note that both apocrine and eccrine sweating occur in the axilla.

cally, are cholinergic when supplying the sweat gland. Within seconds of an appropriate stimulus, eccrine sweat appears on the skin surface, the secretory activity also being heralded by a drop in skin electrical resistance. In the absence of continuous impulses, secretion stops rapidly. Storage of eccrine sweat does not occur. There are no inhibitory nerves to the gland, and sympathectomy results in local anhidrosis in the area supplied.

Heat is the prime stimulus to eccrine sweating, yet emotional stress may produce widespread sweating, especially on the forehead, axillae, palms and soles. Reflex sweating of the face may occur as a result of eating highly spiced foods. Local axon reflexes in the skin may also initiate local sweating. This is to be seen as a peripheral band of sweat droplets around patches of inflammation, particularly on the feet and hands.

Pharmacologically, the gland responds to acetylcholine and pilocarpine. It is inhibited by atropine in relatively large doses. Recently, it has

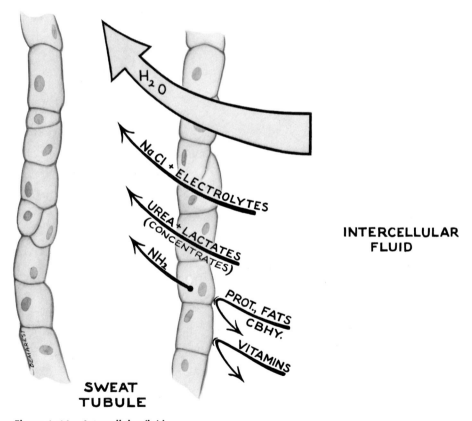

INTERCELLULAR FLUID

SWEAT TUBULE

Figure 1–14.   Intercellular fluid

Diagrammatic representation of the secretory process occurring within the *eccrine* sweat tubule. The prime function of the eccrine sweat gland is to secrete water for evaporative cooling. (PROT., proteins; CBHY., carbohydrates.)

been emphasized that some individuals may show some sweating in response to local epinephrine, but this is not of any known clinical or physiologic significance.

Sweat may be formed in enormous quantities, i.e., as much as several thousand cc. per hour. Its chemical composition has been extensively studied, though it is difficult to obtain sweat in an uncontaminated state. Fundamentally, it is a very dilute saline solution. Carbohydrates, fats and proteins are not found. The constituents present occur either as a result of an osmotic inability to secrete distilled water or as a result of the chemical kinetics of the secretory process itself. In any event, the gland is not an excretory organ comparable to the kidney. All of the electrolytes to be found in plasma or interstitial fluid occur in sweat to a lesser extent. Three compounds, however, are actually concentrated in sweat. These are the lactate ion, urea and ammonia. It is suspected that these reflect intracellular mechanisms responsible for the formation of sweat. The chloride level of sweat shows fluctuations that are related to the degree of acclimatization of the individual to a warm environment. Highly acclimatized persons secrete much less chloride, as do individuals on a low chloride diet. The gland is sensitive to circulating corticosteroids, the chloride excretion falling in the presence of higher steroid levels. Finally, the chemistry of eccrine sweat is a diagnostic tool in mucoviscidosis. Here the chloride levels rise considerably, indicating a defect in sweat gland function, since the most perfectly functioning glands secrete a product most closely resembling distilled water.

CORIUM AND SUBCUTANEOUS TISSUE

Diseases of the skin focus sharply on the epidermis, since this is the site of many distinctive patterns, ranging from the vesiculation of contact dermatitis to common superficial tumors such as superficial nevi, verrucae and epitheliomas. Morphologic dermatologic diagnosis derives in great part from the variegated patterns woven by epidermal changes.

In contrast, the corium or true skin is more hidden and the changes in it harder to interpret on inspection. Biopsy and histologic study are often necessary. The corium is actually the major portion of the skin; it is what we feel as skin. It is simply another of the many fascia in the body and is, thus, the most external of all connective tissue sheaths. Accordingly, it is frequently involved in many diffuse systemic disorders of connective tissue. The ready accessibility of a tremendous expanse of corium often permits an awareness and observation of "collagen" diseases denied one in the other sectors of clinical and laboratory medicine and radiology.

The corium is not a uniquely cutaneous structure. It shows the same age changes as does any connective tissue, the same individual variations, and the same functional differences in various areas. The loose, delicate corium of the infant bears but little resemblance to the hard, firm corium of the prize fighter or to the fine atrophic corium of the octogenarian. Yet, basically, the same three anatomic components are present:

1. Cells
2. Fibers
3. Matrix

Of these, collagen fibers are the overwhelmingly predominant element of normal corium. Just as the stratum corneum is keratin, sebum is lipid and sweat is water, corium is collagen. Throughout these collagen bundles runs a most elaborate system of nerves and lymphatic blood vessels. The corium supports and protects these peripheral networks. Also, as we have already seen, the corium is invaded by the epidermal downgrowths of hair follicles and glands. Functionally, the corium has a major protective role for these varied essential components of skin.

All of the corium derives from the mesodermal ancestor of cells, the primitive mesenchymal cell. This is the reticulum cell, completely unobtrusive in histologic sections of normal adult corium, yet always ready to proliferate and differentiate in times of injury or disease. This stem cell gives rise to the following three normal connective tissue cells:

1. Fibrocyte
2. Histiocyte
3. Mastocyte

The *fibrocyte* is the master cell of the corium, since it forms the fibrous and matrix substance of the corium. Presumably, abnormalities in this cell reflect themselves in the collagen disease pattern. The *histiocyte* is the scavenger or macrophage cell. This cell is part of the reticuloendothelial system and, as such, stands continuously ready to engulf foreign materials. Its phagocytic function may be demonstrated by the injection of dyes or pigments. The *mastocyte* is a specialized cell about the vascular tree and contains considerable quantities of histamine and heparin. Damage to this cell releases the granules of histamine and heparin, with a marked resultant local urticaria and erythema. Considerable overgrowth of these cells produces the uncommon clinical entity urticaria pigmentosa. In this disease, stroking of the affected skin with a blunt object or rubbing of the lesion is followed by an immediate local hive that is rather diagnostic.

The fibrous element of the corium is made up largely of collagen. The second type of fiber, *elastin*, is found in very small amounts. Collagen is a protein; indeed, one of the toughest and most resistant of those made in nature. It is laid down as many white branching fibers that are at once flexible and soft, yet possess great resistance to tensile strain. Early immature collagen may be distinguished histologically (argyrophilic) and, as such, has been called reticulum fiber. Later in the aging process these fibers grow by lateral association to form adult bands of nonbranching collagen. Elastic fibers are single yellow strands that branch and anastomose. They are composed of an elastic type of protein, elastin. These, as well as collagen, are chemically albuminoids. In disease processes, degenerative or

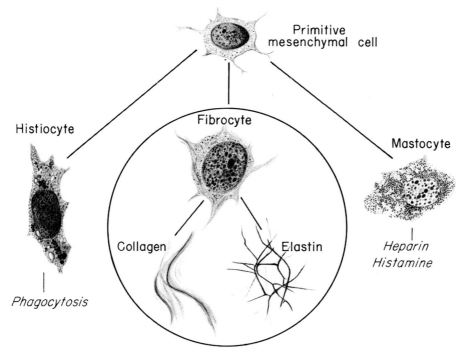

Figure 1–15.   Schematic representation of the "cellular morphogenesis" in normal human skin.

Recent studies indicate a possible mesenchymal origin for the Langerhans cell.

destructive influences may select the collagen or elastin tissues and produce distinctive histologic patterns.

The third main component of the corium is really a ghost structure, the *interfibrillar cement.* It is the ground substance or matrix. It is not seen in ordinary histologic preparations, yet it is chemically characterizable and subject to disease changes. It is largely mucoid, being composed of mucopolysaccharides, such as hyaluronic acid and chondroitin sulfuric acid. Some observers feel that it is secreted by the mast cell, which also forms the closely allied compound heparin. The clinical effect of the enzyme hyaluronidase is a potentiate intracutaneous spreading by temporarily breaking down the barrier of hyaluronic acid, for it is through this milieu that much of the passive intradermal transfer must take place. Enormous changes in the quantity of ground substance are seen in relation to age, since the embryonic skin is predominantly ground substance, whereas, in normal adult tissue it appears to be absent histologically. Much may be learned by further study of this matrix substance and its chemistry in relation to collagen disease.

The subcutaneous tissue is simply another layer of connective tissue, which specializes in the formation of fat. In the corium the fibrocyte is the

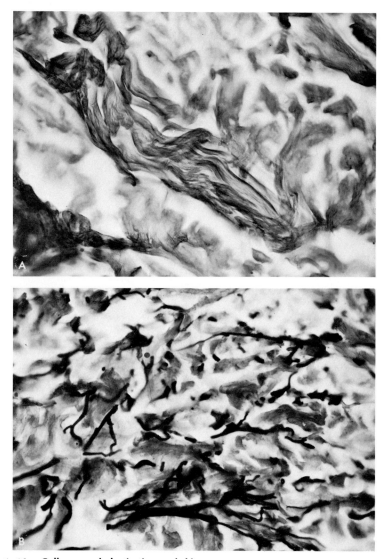

Figure 1–16.   Collagen and elastic tissue of skin

A. Bundles of collagen in normal human dermis. Note wavy character of central strands which have been cut longitudinally. The fibers which have been cut transversely lie on either side. (Magnification 425 ×.)

B. Elastic tissue in normal human dermis. Note the fact that the elastic fibers which have been differentially stained are thin and that they do branch. The small dark fragments are normal elastic fibers which have been cut in cross section. (Magnification 425 ×.)

key cell, forming collagen. In the subcutaneous tissue it is the lipocyte that manufactures and stores such enormous quantities of fat that the whole cytoplasm becomes lipoidal in character. It is also mesodermal in origin. As everyone is aware, individual and area differences in this fat deposition are great. The eyelid lacks significant subcutaneous tissue, while the abdomen may abound in it. Such considerations as these striking area differences in the corium, as well as the subcutaneous tissue, must be taken into account in various disease patterns and in plastic surgery. Actually, the depth of this fat layer is such as to make disease patterns indistinct. Much less is known about the subcutaneous tissue than about the epidermis and corium because of its disadvantageous position from the standpoint of observation and biopsy. The term panniculitis is used glibly but often with far less precision than is the case with epidermal disease patterns.

Functionally, the subcutaneous tissue retains the protective property of connective tissue and also acts as an effective heat insulator. Furthermore, this adipose tissue is a reserve depot of calories to be utilized in periods of starvation.

BLOOD VESSELS AND NERVES

The blood supply is a major independent system within the connective tissue sheaths. To it we owe our nutrition, our cellular and humoral local

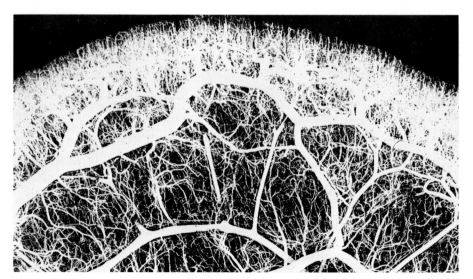

Figure 1–17.   Microangiogram of the tip of a rabbit ear showing the extraordinary vascularity of the skin and also both coarse (macromesh) and fine (micromesh) vascular networks. Micrograph taken with Cosslett-Nixon x-ray projection microscope. (Magnification 10 ×.) (Courtesy of Dr. R. L. de C. H. Saunders, Dalhousie University, Halifax, N.S., Canada.)

defenses and a major portion of our thermal homeostasis. This system, like the connective tissue, is of mesodermal origin and shows a high degree of anatomic as well as functional specialization. The capillary remains the most primitive and undifferentiated. It is here that nutrition and exchange of materials take place. All of the salts and water pass freely, yet most of the plasma protein and all of the erythrocytes remain within the lumen. Injury to any area releases histamine and heparin from the mast cell, with enormous changes occurring in capillary permeability. Protective immune proteins pour out, as well as cells, and local edema ensues. The arterioles and venules of the skin deserve mention. It is the smooth muscle of the arterioles that permits the vasoconstriction so strikingly demonstrable in Raynaud's phenomenon. Unfortunately, skin color changes are not readily transformable into simple hemodynamic formulae. The complicating features of depth and location of the vessel, as well as its size, must be considered. Basically, however, the color of skin reflects the subcapillary venous supply, its flow and the degree of oxygenation.

Arteriovenous anastomoses are a striking feature of the skin of the extremities. These A-V shunts, termed glomera are of considerable importance in heat regulation. Anatomically, they are distinctive. They may occasionally overgrow, producing a painful lesion, the glomus tumor.

All of the blood vessels of the skin are under the same humoral and neural influences that are operative elsewhere in the body, though at times the skin response may be paradoxical. Circulating epinephrine may trigger the blanching of generalized vasoconstriction. Circulating serotonin has been shown to produce blotchy vasodilation and flushing, as in the malignant carcinoid syndrome. The neural control is mediated through the sympathetic nervous system, and central as well as local influences abound. The axon reflex is a striking vascular response in the skin in which the central pathways are not necessary. It is seen most regularly in the triple response of Lewis and accounts, in part, for the marked vasodilation seen in all types of dermatitic skin. To elicit Lewis' response, one strokes normal skin firmly with a blunt object. Within 15 seconds a red line develops in the exact area of trauma. This is due to the release of histamine from the mastocytes, causing local dilation of the arterioles. It is independent of all nervous control and reflects the powerful vaso-effects of histamine. Shortly thereafter the second response appears. This is an erythema spreading out from the site of trauma. This is the axon reflex that results from stimulation of the sensory nerves with local reflex discharges causing vasodilation. The local nerves must be intact for eliciting this response, since local anesthetics eliminate this axon reflex. Finally, the third response of Lewis is manifest within several minutes. This is the wheal, or local urticaria, caused by the outpouring of fluids from the capillaries that have been affected by the histamine released originally.

Although acetylcholine causes vasodilation, no vasodilator nerves are known to exist in the skin. All of the neural influences are believed to stem from adrenergic vasoconstrictive impulses over the sympathetic fibers.

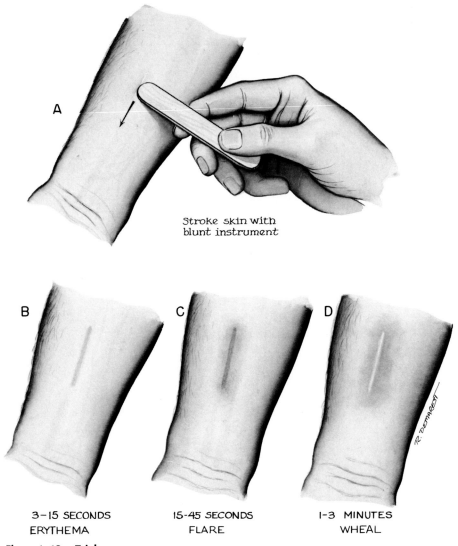

Stroke skin with
blunt instrument

| 3–15 SECONDS | 15-45 SECONDS | 1-3 MINUTES |
| ERYTHEMA | FLARE | WHEAL |

Figure 1–18. Triple response

Diagrammatic representation of the triple response of Lewis. Mechanical injury of the skin invariably leads to the above sequence of vascular changes.

Direct physical phenomena often influence the skin markedly. Very slight mechanical trauma may cause blanching, and cold may also cause vasoconstriction by stimulation of the smooth muscular wall of the arteriole. Local heating, conversely, produces vasodilation. Local pH and carbon dioxide changes are also operative. It becomes evident that the blood supply of the skin is under highly complex interrelated influences that deny any simple formulation.

The lymphatic system of the skin is an auxiliary circulatory system. Throughout the skin are two major plexuses of blind, thin, endothelial lymphatics. This is a primitive system representing an alternate pathway to the venous channels. It is sluggish and not directly responsive to neural or pharmacologic stimuli. Its role in skin disease, other than in reducing edema, is minor or unrecognized.

The nerve supply to the skin is one of the most vital of all its structures. Here we find the system for motor control of glands and vessels as well as the vast sentient end organs so critical in local and general protection from noxious agents. The motor system courses through the skin as the efferent sympathetic fibers. Both cholinergic and adrenergic, they supply various structures. The adrenergic fibers activate the arrectores pilorum, arteriolar vasoconstriction and the contraction of the apocrine myoepithelium resulting in apocrine sweating. The cholinergic fibers supply the eccrine sweat gland (Fig. 1–19). It should be remembered that the epidermis itself, the hair follicle and the sebaceous gland are not under neural control. Further-

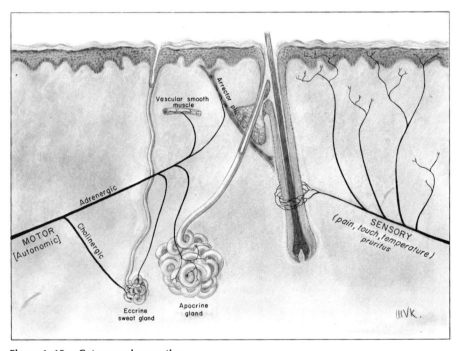

Figure 1–19. Cutaneous innervation

Diagrammatic representation of cutaneous innervation. The skin is supplied by motor (autonomic) nerves and by sensory (spinal) nerves. The cholinergic division of the motor nerve activates the secretory cells of the eccrine sweat gland. The adrenergic component of the motor system activates the myoepithelium of apocrine and eccrine glands and the smooth muscle of the arteriole and arrector pili. The sebaceous gland is not innervated by motor nerves. Generally, the sensory nerve endings are free, unorganized branches. It is only in areas such as the palms and soles that the "specialized" nerve endings are found.

more, trophic fibers to the skin are unknown, as are inhibitory fibers. All of the efferent nerves supplying the skin are stimulatory.

The cutaneous nerves possess a full complement of afferent sensory as well as motor nerves. These are the fibers that conduct the impulses giving rise to the skin sensations of pruritus, pain, touch and temperature. They may be small (unmyelinated) or large (myelinated), and their termini may be undifferentiated or may appear as highly organized sensory nerve endings. Actually, the palm and sole are among the few places in which such specialized nerve endings occur. Present beliefs in neurophysiology are shifting away from the concept that the specificity of sensation is determined by highly specialized receptors. The former teaching of a special end organ for each sensation (Meissner's, Pacini's, tactile; Krause's, cold; Ruffini's, heat) is being abandoned. In its place has come the concept that spatial and temporal relationships in stimuli firing of the nerve are critical. One group holds that certain fiber size relationships are evident, but this is not universally believed.

The fine sensory network courses through the corium and, until recently, was thought not to enter the epidermis. Convincing evidence, however, of free nerve endings within the epidermis has become available, and these are exquisitely attuned to superficial changes in temperature or pressure. They also sense many chemical changes in the epidermis as well as in the dermis. Touch (including its analogue, tickle) and temperature sense are of lesser importance in disease states. Pain and pruritus are of much greater clinical significance. Pain has been defined by many descriptive terms, but basically one perceives two types, the *sharp prick pain* and the *dull aching or burning pain*. Neurophysiologic studies suggest that sharp pain is mediated by impulses passing rapidly up the large medullated fibers, whereas burning pain is associated with slow impulses on fine unmyelinated fibers. This distinction is valid in general terms, although, as in all biology, not absolute. Any type of injury to the skin will initiate pain. The prick of the hypodermic needle, the heat of the electrodesiccating needle or the chemical effect of an alcohol on dermatitic skin — all fire the pain fibers. At times the impulse passage may be blocked by actual destruction (phenol), or reversible anesthesia (procaine) or cooling (ethyl chloride spray) of the peripheral nerve. It is pertinent to note again here that the normal skin, unlike the mucosa, cannot be anesthetized by topical application of local anesthetics. Only in denuded skin does this occur, and there irregularly.

Itching is a uniquely cutaneous symptom. Pain may develop in any organ, but itching is a distinctive, at times maddening, sensation associated with most forms of dermatitis and many other conditions. The urge to claw, scratch, dig or excoriate is the main reason for many patients seeking medical advice. Itching may be incessant, crippling and demanding. It varies in degree with different people. Unquestionably, some are "itchish," and for these patients contact dermatitis, scabies and lichen planus, for instance, are major evils. Others, fortunately, fail to perceive or develop significant pruritus, despite the presence of diseases that are commonly pruritogenic. In some patients, marked itching may occur in the absence of any gross or microscopic change.

Recent studies have demonstrated that pruritus arises as a result of a distinctive pattern of stimulation of the fine subepidermal nerve network. This pattern of stimulation is provided for by proteolytic enzymes. These proteinases are released from the epidermis as a result of either primary irritation or allergic sensitization reactions. Other sources include the blood and cellular infiltrates, as well as the surface bacterial and fungal flora. Trace amounts may be adequate, and in the pruritic lichenified skin of atopic dermatitis, these enzymes act in a dilution of over one to a million. The same small unmyelinated nerves that subserve burning pain act for pruritus. Indeed, as the stimulus increases in intensity, the sensation may become a burning itch or burning alone. Clinically, it is commonly recognized that burning and pruritus are allied sensations.

Methods that interrupt pain will also interrupt pruritus. Local anesthetics, cold and sectioning of the peripheral nerve or anterior cordotomy all eliminate both pain and pruritus. Sympathectomy has no effect. It is significant to note that damage of the subepidermal network abolishes itch selectively, since deep receptors do not exist for this sensation as they do for pain. Accordingly, severe dermatitic skin may not itch simply because of inflammatory damage to the itch receptor. With healing and regeneration of the network, the pruritus may once again develop. Many of the home remedies of the patient for relief of itching (e.g., steaming hot water) are unknowingly based on the principle of damage to the nerve receptor system. It is regrettable that not a single *consistently* effective systemic antipruritic compound has been developed as yet. The methods for relieving pain are much more reliable and efficient than those for relieving itch.

Basic Pathologic Patterns | 2

The skin has a rather limited range of reaction patterns that may, however, express themselves in widely varying clinical syndromes. It may react with a functional change or an inflammatory or proliferative one. The great diversity of clinical portraits results from the fact that the skin is composed of thirteen distinct units. Meld with this the great individual, area and age differences, and an exceedingly complex gallery results. These patterns may be further masked by the effects of external treatment, well or poorly selected. Much of this diversity is due to the fact that the opportunity to view the pathologic process, both gross and microscopic, in the skin is much greater than in the case of most internal organs. Disease changes in the skin have been "overdescribed"; and a surfeit of observations, by general medical standards, has resulted. In order to resolve some of this confusion it is necessary to hold fast to simple basic concepts. By analogy, one must still perceive the common phenomenon of fire in a lighted match, an explosion, a pile of smoking leaves or the launching blast of a satellite. The singular basic facts about any eruption must be perceived: Is it one of function, of inflammation or of growth? Which unit of the skin is primarily involved? To answer these questions is the goal of diagnosis. In this book we are concerned with the significant, the common, and the following outline will aid in correlating the clinical with the basic pathologic processes. Only the common problems will be specifically cited.

CELLULAR ALTERATIONS

Keratinocyte

A. Alteration in Function. The function of the keratinocyte is to elaborate a protective protein covering, the stratum corneum. The corn and the callus present striking functional changes (hyperkeratosis) due to stimulation of the epidermis by intermittent pressure. In ichthyosis there is a decreased rate of sloughing of the stratum corneum, with resultant thickening of the horny layer. Focal changes are also seen at the follicular orifices in acne. Here the functional change becomes evident as a comedo (blackhead).

47

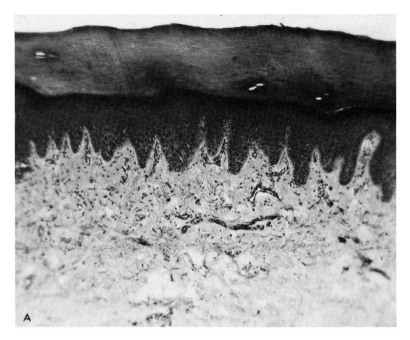

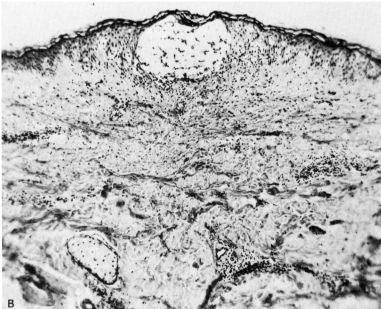

Figure 2–1. *A.* Alteration in function of the keratinocyte (epidermal cell). Note the enormous surface deposition of keratin occurring as a result of keratinocyte activity. In this slide the keratinocyte is also showing some benign proliferative change. This is hyperkeratosis. (Magnification 70×.)

B. Alteration from injury to keratinocyte (epidermal cell). Note clear space in the epidermis which is a vesicle resulting from destruction of keratinocytes following an allergic reaction. This is an example of contact dermatitis. (Magnification 70×.)

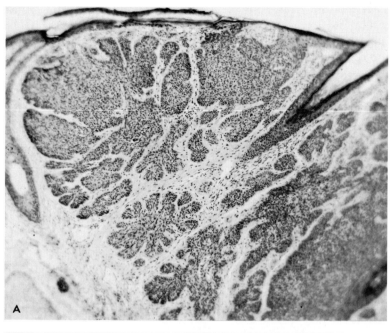

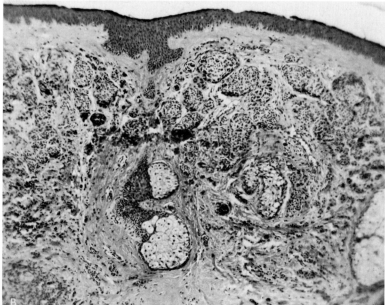

Figure 2–2.   *A.* Alteration in growth of keratinocyte (epidermal cell). In this slide the keratinocyte is showing an enormous proliferative change, so that the epidermal cells have invaded the entire corium. This is a basal cell epithelioma. (Magnification 70 ×.)

B. Alteration in growth of melanocyte. Here the melanocyte has shown a malignant proliferative growth change. Clusters of malignant melanocytes are seen throughout the dermis. The keratinocytes are normal. This is a malignant melanoma. (Magnification 70 ×.)

B. Alteration from Injury. Damage to the keratinocyte is the cause of a major portion of all the disturbances seen in the skin. This is the principal pathologic site of all forms of dermatitis. The cell change may be morphologically slight, producing only the secondary changes of erythema in the nerve and vascular rete below, or it may assume the form of massive collections of fluid within the epidermis. This is the elementary unitary response of the keratinocyte to chemical, thermal, radiant or mechanical trauma. Thus, the gross changes in a dermatitis may do little to disclose its cause. The bulla of a thermal burn duplicates the bulla of poison ivy dermatitis. Again, viruses may cause the dermatitis (herpes, varicella, zoster, variola). Pemphigus and the other bullous diseases also find their basic pathologic pattern in the keratinocyte.

C. Alteration in Growth. Verrucae and seborrheic keratoses are the simplest examples of common benign overgrowth of the keratinocyte. Basal and squamous cell epitheliomas are the common malignancies involving the keratinocyte. Intermediate or premalignant growths of the keratinocyte are also common. These are the senile keratoses of the exposed areas of skin and leukoplakia of the mucous membranes.

Melanocyte

A. Alteration in Function. This is common. Hyperfunction is seen in tanning, chloasma and freckles. By contrast, loss of pigment formation is seen as vitiligo.

B. Alteration from Injury. As in A.

C. Alteration in Growth. This is probably the most common benign growth change in the skin. One must recognize that the nevus cell, which composes the pigmented part of the common nevus (mole), is the melanocyte. This is a benign process. In contrast, one sometimes, though fortunately *rarely*, sees malignant change in the melanocyte. When it occurs, it produces the malignant melanoma, one of the most dangerous and unpredictable of all tumors.

Fibrocyte

A. Alteration in Function. Scar and keloid formation are examples of increase in function, whereas the atrophy of age is a sign of functional involution of the cell.

B. Alteration from Injury. As in A.

C. Alteration in Growth. Rare (fibromas).

Histiocyte

A. Alteration in Function. This is the macrophage cell, which appears in all granulomas (syphilis, tuberculosis, leprosy, sarcoidosis and the deep mycoses).

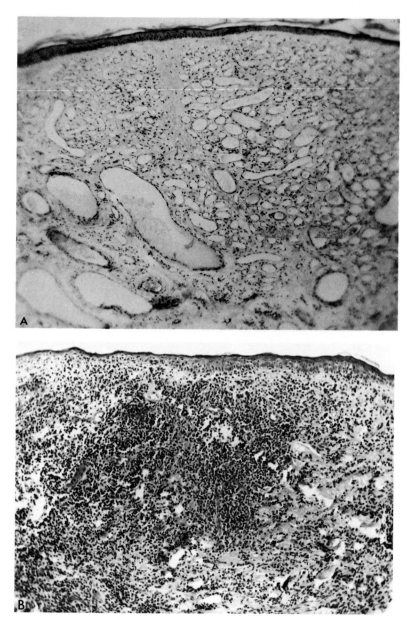

Figure 2–3.   *A.* Alterations in growth of vascular tissue. The dermis is filled with vascular channels. This is a capillary hemangioma. (Magnification 70 ×.)

B. Alterations in growth of extraneous cells. The dermis is solidly packed with myeloid cells. This is the picture seen in leukemia cutis. (Magnification 100 ×.)

B. Alteration from Injury.   As in A.
C. Alteration in Growth.   As in A.

Mastocyte

Rare. Principally mastocytosis (urticaria pigmentosa).

Lipocyte

Rare.

Myeloid-lymphoid Cells

Found in inflammatory lesions of skin (benign and malignant).

Schwann Cells

Rare (neuromas and neurofibromas).

GLANDULAR ALTERATIONS

Sebaceous Gland

A. Alteration in Function.   Hyperfunction occurs and is known as seborrhea.
B. Alteration from Injury.   Rare.
C. Alteration in Growth.   Normal increased activity at puberty. In acne, a sebaceous gland may undergo pressure atrophy as a result of poral occlusion and concomitant cyst formation.

Apocrine Sweat Gland

Here the significant aberration is bacterial infection known as hidradenitis suppurativa.

Eccrine Sweat Gland

The primary pathologic change here is poral occlusion with resultant sweat retention, which triggers a variable picture (miliaria).

ADDITIONAL ALTERATIONS

Hair Follicle

A. Alteration in Function.   Failure to grow hair (hereditary alopecia, alopecia areata) is the common alteration in function. The converse is hirsutism.

B. Alteration from Injury.   Destruction of the entire follicle by external factors (burns, hot comb alopecia) or by inflammatory reaction (lupus erythematosus). Damage or partial destruction may lead to ingrown hairs and secondary inflammatory changes (pili incarnati following close shaving).

C. Alteration in Growth.   Uncommon (congenital hairy nevi, trichoepithelioma).

Vascular System

The growth change of the hemangioma is the chief alteration here.

Nerve Tissue

Rare.

REFERENCES

Lever, W. F.: Histopathology of the Skin. 5th ed. J. B. Lippincott Co., Philadelphia, 1975.

Montgomery, H.: Dermatopathology, 2 Vols. Hoeber Medical Division, Harper and Row, New York, 1966.

Plewig, G., and Kligman, A. M.: Acne: Morphogenesis and Treatment. Springer-Verlag, New York, 1975.

3 | Dermatologic Diagnosis

EXAMINATION OF THE SKIN

Careful inspection of the skin should be a part of any complete physical examination. Adequate lighting and exposure of all involved areas of skin are necessary if proper identification of the principal types of lesions is to be made and the distribution patterns recognized. The morphology of the lesions and these patterns suggest a number of differential diagnostic possibilities.

Lesions

Macules. Circumscribed variations in color of the skin. Of these, acute erythematous macules and purpura are the most important, particularly in terms of systemic disease and drug reactions. Other types include melanin pigment, e.g., flat moles and freckles; and extrinsically derived pigment, e.g., tattoos.

Papules and Papulosquamous Lesions. Papules are raised circumscribed lesions of the skin, of varying color and other physical characteristics. They range in size from as small as 1 to 2 mm. in diameter to much larger. At a greater size, whether through enlargement of single lesions or coalescence with others, the lesions become plaques. If papular lesions extend deeply into the skin, they are commonly called nodules or tumors.

Listed below are some common and other uncommon to rare skin diseases that begin as papules (tumors of skin excluded).

COMMON*

Acne — grade I	Discoid lupus erythematosus
Psoriasis	Cysts — many types
Pityriasis rosea (usually macular)	Leprosy (in endemic areas)
Secondary syphilis	Angiomas — cherry, spider
Insect bites (many varieties) usually urticarial at onset	Anthrax — initially
	Callus
Lichen planus	Lichenification and scratch papules
Keratoses — actinic and seborrheic	Milia

UNCOMMON

Fibrous papule of nose
Hodgkin's disease
Lymphangioma
Lymphoma
Mastocytosis
Necrobiosis lipoidica diabeticorum
  (early)

Neurofibromatosis (with pigmented
  macules)
Parapsoriasis
Polymorphic light eruption
Prurigo nodularis
Reiter's syndrome
Sarcoidosis
Swimming pool granuloma

---

*The description of various diseases listed as common and uncommon here and subsequently is based on the authors' clinical experience over several decades. The order in which diseases are listed is a rough reflection of their prevalence in a temperate climate. In a hot, humid climate the order changes. Superficial infections of all types, for example, will be seen with much greater frequency than in temperate climates.

Plaques. Ordinarily result from a coalescence of papules. Any raised scaling lesion larger than 2 or 3 cm. is usually so termed. Plaques may be very large, such as those located on the lower back and buttocks in psoriasis.

Nodules and Tumors. *Nodules* are characterized by palpable subcutaneous or superficial lesions of varying consistency and size. Lesions of more than 2 cm. in diameter are usually termed *tumors*, although this distinction is not clear-cut. There may be no color change if the skin itself is not involved, but should the skin be involved, its color may be erythematous, purplish, brownish yellow or blue (as in blue nevus). Nodules are sometimes preliminary evidence of infection extending from an underlying focus or a primary inoculation syndrome.

Nodules may persist for months or years without change, and these are ordinarily harmless. In nodules that appear or enlarge suddenly, malignant disease may be present, and biopsy and a general medical survey become mandatory. Nodules often progress to ulceration.

Nodules or tumors may be a conspicuous feature at some time during the course of the following diseases. Ultra-rare diseases are not included, but in some cases, e.g., onchocerciasis, the disease may be widespread in one geographic area (Africa) but unknown in others.

COMMON

Acne
Adenopathy
Carcinoma — many types
Cherry hemangioma
Cutaneous leishmaniasis
Erythema nodosum
Fibroma
Foreign body granuloma
Ganglion

Keloid
Hypertrophic scars
Leprosy (in endemic areas)
Mucoid cyst
Neurofibromatosis
Prurigo nodularis
Pyogenic granuloma
Rheumatic nodules
Xanthoma tuberosum

UNCOMMON

Actinomycosis
Bromoderma
Calcinosis cutis
Erythema induratum
Fat necrosis
Gumma
Hodgkin's disease
Iododerma
Lupus vulgaris

Nevoxanthoendothelioma
Nevus sebaceus
Primary cutaneous blastomycosis
Swimming pool granuloma
Urticaria pigmentosum
Glomus tumor
Kaposi's tumor
Sarcoidosis
Gouty tophi
Lymphoma

Wheals (Hives).   A special type of papule or plaque, consisting of white to pinkish edema of the skin, with or without surrounding erythema. The process may be evanescent and relatively inconsequential, e.g., a few insect bites, or it may be systemically significant, e.g., penicillin reaction.

Vesicles, Pustules and Bullae.   *Vesicles* are superficial, distinct lesions of the skin containing serum, which is sometimes tinged with blood. *Bullae* are larger similar lesions, usually so termed if more than 1 to 2 cm. in diameter. *Pustules* are essentially vesicles that contain pus. Microorganisms are frequently demonstrable from them, but they are occasionally sterile, e.g., pustular psoriasis.

None of these lesions remain intact very long. They soon evolve into crusts or superficial erosions, or become secondarily infected. The general medical significance of this group varies widely. Vesicles resulting from a contact sensitization reaction or moderate physical forces heal within a few days to two weeks unless mistreated, traumatized by scratching or complicated by secondary infection.

Chronic or recurrent bullous dermatoses may be life threatening and deserve the most searching investigation and adequate treatment.

COMMON VESICLES

Herpes simplex
Contact dermatitis
Sunburn
Acute fungal infections
Nummular dermatitis

Drug eruptions
"Id" reactions
Herpes zoster
Pompholyx
Hand, foot and mouth disease

UNCOMMON VESICLES

Benign familial chronic pemphigus
Dermatitis herpetiformis

COMMON BULLAE

Impetigo

Drug Eruptions

Contact Dermatitis

Erythema multiforme

Friction response

UNCOMMON BULLAE

Blister beetle bite

Dermatitis herpetiformis

Diphtheria cutis

Epidermolysis bullosa

Erysipelas (sometimes)

Fogo selvagem (South American

   pemphigus)

Herpes gestationis

Pemphigoid

Pemphigus

Toxic epidermal necrolysis

COMMON PUSTULES

Impetigo

Secondary infections (pyoderma)

Acute candidiasis

Nummular dermatitis

Varicella

UNCOMMON PUSTULES

Kaposis varicelliform eruption

Subcorneal pustular eruption

Certain distinctive types of skin lesions occur in the evolution of the basic skin disease. These include:

Scales. Scales vary greatly in their appearance, abundance and adhesiveness. A few are so characteristic as to have some diagnostic significance. *Psoriasis,* in chronic plaque form, presents a silvery-white to gray appearance that is highly characteristic. The scales are resistant to removal but when scraped off, reveal tiny bleeding points from the capillary loops (Auspitz sign), which are fairly typical but not diagnostic.

In many patients with *seborrheic dermatitis,* the scales have a yellowish, greasy appearance. This is especially apparent in some patients with Parkinson's disease. The scaling in *ichthyosis* may be dry and diffuse and, particularly on the lower legs, may assume a fish scale-like lamellar appearance, especially in a cold environment. Lesions of pityriasis rosea and tinea corporis tend to scale principally at the margin of the individual lesions.

Ulcers. Ulcerative destruction of the skin and subcutaneous tissue obviously reflects a potent force. The causes are extraordinarily numerous and often mixed and sometimes defy precise detection. The following listing indicates the chief etiologic factors that may be operative.

1. Traumatic — mechanical, heat and cold, electrical, chemical, neurotropic and radiological (usually late).

2. Microbiologic — An extraordinarily diverse list including various types of bacterial, viral and fungal infections and parasitic infestations. A striking feature in the past decade, coincident with exposure of the general population to more and different antibiotics, has been the recognition of ulceration produced by organisms rarely encountered or recognized in the past as productive of clinical diseases. Patients on immunosuppressive therapy are particularly vulnerable.

3. Tumors of many types.

4. Factitial — Often escaping detection for years.

5. Systemic disease — The so-called vasculitic ulcers, e.g., ulcerative colitis, rheumatoid arthritis and lupus erythematosus.

6. Stasis—Lymphatic and venous and atherosclerosis, especially in diabetes.

Crusts. Dried accumulation of serum, pus and applied medications on the skin vary widely in appearance. The important thing is to determine what is underneath, e.g., dermatitis, superficial infection or ulcer. Of all crusted lesions, those of impetigo, herpes simplex, zoster-varicella and ecthyma are the most characteristic.

Scars. Connective tissue replacement of skin and subcutaneous tissue obviously result most frequently from a previous ulcerative process. In new scars it is important to determine whether or not there is a temporarily hypertrophic or progressive keloidal tendency in the lesion, because much can be accomplished by intralesional corticosteroid therapy. Certain scar-like conditions, e.g., localized scleroderma, arise sui generis without previous ulcerative change. Discoid lupus erythematosus produces characteristic scarring ringed by an active border, dilated follicles and sometimes telangiectasia.

Configuration of Lesions

Certain arrangements of lesions are highly suggestive diagnostically. Examples include:

Grouped. Lesions in herpes simplex and zoster occur in groups.

Annular. Almost always in pityriasis rosea, tinea corporis and tinea cruris. Sometimes in secondary syphilis (especially in Blacks), psoriasis, lichen planus and erythema multiforme. Some granulomas, e.g., sarcoid and granuloma annulare.

Linear. Arrangement of lesions in a precise line may be seen in warts, lichen planus, psoriasis and contact dermatitis. A roughly linear distribution is characteristic of herpes zoster and some primary inoculation syndromes. e.g., sporotrichosis.

Distribution Patterns of Lesions

Another significant aid to dermatologic diagnosis is the manner in which the lesions are distributed to various parts of the skin surface and to the mucous membranes. Though none of the following patterns is absolutely constant, the typical distribution is highly suggestive.

Acne.   Face, neck, upper chest and back. In explosive "tropical" acne, the lesions may become much more extensive and inflammatory.

Atopic Dermatitis.   The pattern is very constant in young adults, less so in infants and the middle-aged. Antecubital and popliteal spaces, face, neck, wrists and hands. This is potentially a very disabling and unpredictable disease.

Contact Dermatitis.   Areas exposed to the environment or to particular components of clothing or accessories.

Erythema Multiforme.   Hands, feet, elbows and knees and mucous membranes. In severe cases the distribution may be much more extensive, with conjunctival and orificial involvement.

Erythema Nodosum.   Anterior lower legs.

Lichen Planus.   Flexor surface of wrists, male genitalia, mucous surfaces of mouth and vagina, trunk and lower legs.

Lupus Erythematosus (Chronic Discoid).
Cheeks, bridge of nose, scalp and ears.

Seborrheic Dermatitis.   Scalp, portions of face, especially nasolabial folds, eyebrows and occasionally lid margins (blepharitis) and intertriginous areas such as retroauricular, inframammary, axillary and inguinal skin.

Pityriasis Rosea.   Trunk and upper portion of extremities (about 75 per cent of all cases).

Psoriasis.   Elbows, knees, scalp, back, nails and anogenital region.

Photosensitivity Reactions.   Areas exposed to sunlight. May be confused with reaction to environmental contactants, particularly airborne ones.

Scabies.   Male genitalia, between fingers, palms, wrists, axillary folds and female breast areola. Almost never on the face.

HISTORY

The best medical history obviously should include a retrospective record of the patient's genetic background, his past state of health, his reactions to physical and mental stress and to his environment, his sensitivity to oral and parenteral medication and a wide variety of other factors. Many changes in the skin can be interpreted very quickly; in others the most searching inquiry may be necessary.

Certain special aspects of the medical history are of particular importance in interpreting a dermatologic disease in which the possible etiologic factors are not immediately apparent. The following questions represent a practical check list:

1. Any systemic signs or symptoms?
2. Any drugs, systemic or topical?

3. Any unusual exposure to environmental conditions — plants, insects, leeches, heat or cold and sunlight — unusual exposure to warm or cold moisture, recent transfer from geographic areas of endemic disease, unusual special occupations?

4. Any venereal contacts?

5. Any psychosomatic factors, particularly an impulse to perpetuate chronic disease?

6. Any epidemic disease in family or associates?

7. The progression of the eruption since onset: acute, chronic or relapsing? Previous treatment and its effect. Any ionizing radiation?

8. Any seasonal recurrence or evidence of atopy, e.g., hay fever, asthma, rhinitis?

9. Any factors that aggravate symptoms or objective signs? Any improvement when away from work or home?

The family history is not commonly helpful in the initial assessment of a dermatosis. In diseases that remain obscure, however, genetic clues may emerge in a wide variety of skin changes, many of which are rare. The more common include psoriasis, atopic dermatitis, ichthyosis and acne. The true nature of an unusual tendency to develop blisters or large keratoses at sites of pressure on the feet may become apparent from the family history. Aberrations of hair or nail growth are commonly genetic in origin. Patients with vitiligo or alopecia areata sometimes have a family history of these obvious diseases. Many unusual nevoid changes may be interpreted more adequately on the basis of knowledge of the familial background.

SPECIAL DIAGNOSTIC PROCEDURES

In obscure diseases affecting the skin, the entire diagnostic facilities of a general hospital may sometimes have to be involved to arrive at a tenable diagnosis. In practice, it is particularly important to select those special diagnostic procedures that are essential and most likely to yield useful information, because they may involve dislocation of the patient and considerable expense. Performance of almost every test known to medicine requires little diagnostic acumen; initial performance of those likely to be rewarding does.

In addition to standard routine laboratory procedures, the following diagnostic aids are useful in the interpretation of selected dermatoses.

Darkfield Examination.   Thus is indicated in any new ulcerative lesion with an associated bubo, usually in the genital region but sometimes located elsewhere. Warning: few practitioners and laboratory technicians have had adequate experience in the performance of this procedure, but fluorescent staining methods applied to simple dried smears may shortly become available.

Direct Examination.   Examine scales from lesions suspected of being fungal in origin. Cultures may be of interest but are usually not necessary. This procedure is often carried out in conjunction with Wood's light examination.

Wood's Light Examination.   Used for the detection of tinea capitis (in children), tinea versicolor or erythrasma. These two procedures often provide a very rapid and accurate classification of inflammatory processes involving the feet or the anogenital region, with clear indication of the particular treatment most likely to be effective.

Patch Tests.   Extensive testing of this type is rarely feasible in general practice except when a few contactants, e.g., insect repellent or a plant are suspected. Severe reactions may result if the tests are conducted by persons inexperienced in such studies.*

Bacterial Cultures.   It is essential that adequate sampling be done, particularly in chronic lesions that may have relatively little exudate and a mixed flora. A common technical error is to allow the swabs to dry out before they reach the plate or broth.

Biopsy.   This is an essential procedure in many chronic conditions, particularly tumors, some ulcers and granulomas.

Cytologic Smears.   Used in pemphigus, herpes simplex, molluscum contagiosum and suspected tumors of the mouth.

Immunofluorescence.   This histopathologic technique may be very helpful in the differential diagnosis of bullous diseases.

---

*For an exhaustive text on contact dermatitis the reader is referred to Fisher, A. A.: Contact Dermatitis, Lea & Febiger, Philadelphia, 1973.

4 | Dermatoses Affecting the Head and Neck

Two anatomic features of the head and neck are principal contributors to the diseases affecting this region: sebaceous glands and hair. Under ordinary circumstances, the face and neck receive greater amounts of sunlight than any other portion of the body, with resultant high incidence of photogenic reactions, degenerative changes and basal and squamous cell cancer. With modern cosmetic practices, the potentials for contact dermatitis, particularly in women, are numerous.

Although the face is ordinarily subjected to frequent close inspection, some lesions, particularly tumors, often escape early detection in areas in and behind the external ears, the nasal folds, eyelid margins and hairy portions of the scalp. Some common diseases, such as psoriasis, tend to avoid the face but often involve the scalp.

The following diseases may be considered:

COMMON

Acne
Seborrheic dermatitis
Impetigo
Folliculitis
Furuncle
Contact dermatitis
Atopic dermatitis
Alopecia
Keratoses — actinic and seborrheic
Basal cell epithelioma

Squamous cell carcinoma
Melanocytic nevi
Photosensitivity reactions
Rosacea
Angiomas
Perlèche
Senile sebaceous adenoma
Colloid degeneration
Drug reactions
Psoriasis
Urticaria

UNCOMMON

Leishmaniasis cutis*
Pellagra
Radiodermatitis
Sarcoidosis
Secondary syphilis

Syringoma
Systemic sclerosis
Various granulomas
Warts — particularly flat warts
Lupus erythematosus
Keloids

---

*Common in the eastern Mediterranean.

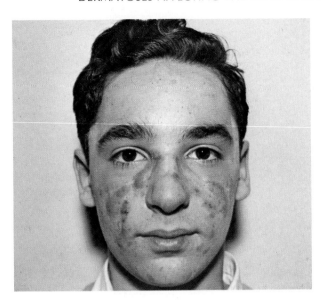

Figure 4–1. Acne

By far the most common disease appearing on the face. In this patient, fluctuant low-grade abscesses appeared suddenly during a prolonged spell of hot humid weather. The response to prolonged low-dosage tetracycline therapy was gratifying, though this is not always the case.

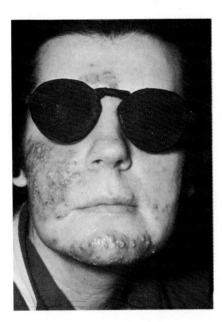

Figure 4–2. Rosacea

Sometimes called acne rosacea. A flushing reaction affecting principally the cheeks, nose and forehead sometimes with associated inflamed papules and pustules. Of cosmetic significance only, except when complicated by rosacea keratitis. Marked telangiectasia and thickening of the skin may develop, particularly on the nose.

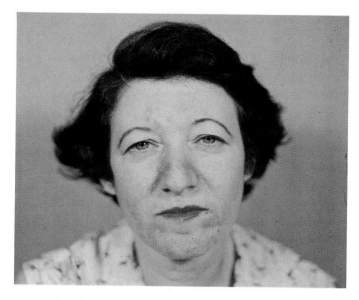

Figure 4–3. Seborrheic dermatitis

Characteristic involvement of forehead, eyebrows, nasal folds and chin. Sometimes occurs in a "butterfly" distribution that may be confused with lupus erythematosus or photosensitivity.

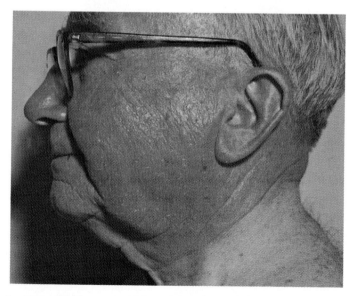

Figure 4–4. Dermatitis due to sensitivity to after-shaving lotion

There was an element of induced photosensitivity as well. Note sharp margination of the dermatitis at the collar line.

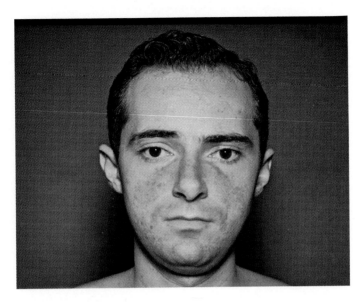

Figure 4–5. Polymorphous light eruption

A relatively common condition which appears to have increased considerably in incidence in the past decade. The differentiation from seborrheic dermatitis or lupus erythematosus is sometimes difficult.

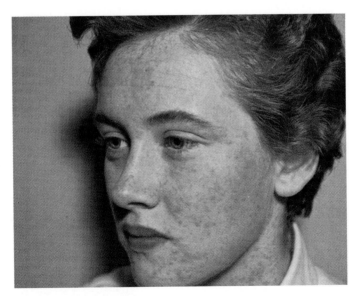

Figure 4–6. Rubella-like drug eruption

This drug eruption, resembling German measles, appeared a few days after the initiation of systemic novobiocin (Cathomycin) therapy. This reaction occurs with disconcerting frequency with this antibiotic. Its use has been abandoned, but other antibiotics may have the same effect.

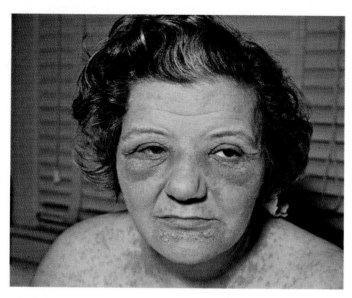

Figure 4–7.   Penicillin reaction

Urticarial and oozing dermatitis lesions appearing within a few hours after injection of the drug. In a patient who has sustained a reaction of this severity, re-administration would carry a high risk of anaphylactic reaction.

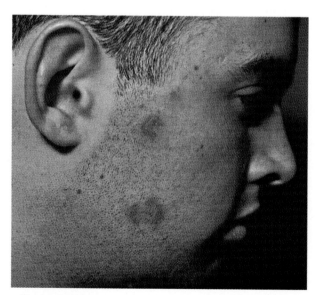

Figure 4–8.   Impetigo contagiosa

Although this mixed streptococcal and staphylococcal infection is superficial, short-term systemic antibiotic therapy is often indicated. Benzathine penicillin, cloxacillin, dicloxacillin or erythromycin are preferred.

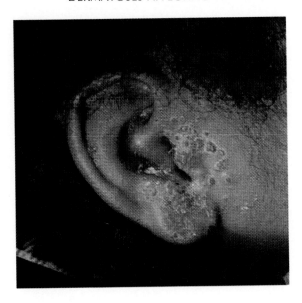

Figure 4–9. Otitis externa with secondary impetiginous infection

Topical cleansing and systemic antibiotic therapy indicated. Suppurative middle-ear infection should be ruled out. There may also be an underlying seborrheic or atopic dermatitis.

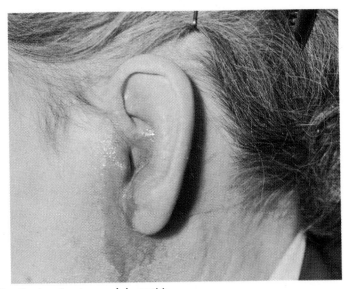

Figure 4–10. Oozing streptococcal dermatitis

Note that extension downward has occurred from dripping of infectious exudate. Systemic therapy as for impetigo. Rule out middle-ear infection.

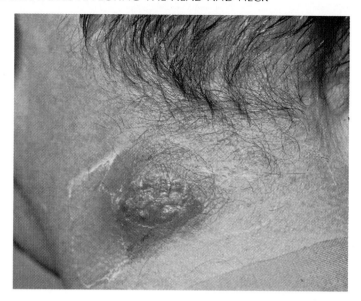

Figure 4–11.   Carbuncle, a collection of furuncles (boils) in a favorite site on the posterior neck

Caused by coagulase-positive *Staphylococcus aureus,* frequently penicillin resistant, especially in infections acquired in the hospital. May be of very serious significance in aged or debilitated patients.

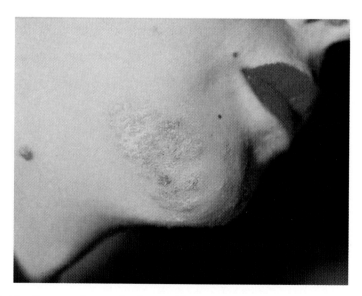

Figure 4–12.   Recurrent herpes simplex ("cold sore") of unusual severity

The vesicles are always grouped. There is no satisfactory preventive or therapeutic means of control. New attacks are precipitated by a wide variety of stresses, including upper respiratory infections and exposure to sunlight.

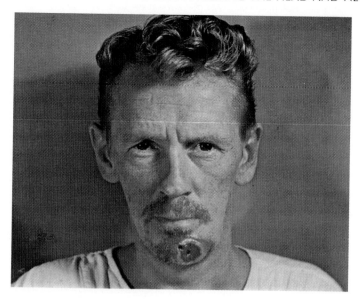

Figure 4–13.   Large extragenital chancre

The treponema of syphilis by no means gain entrance only through the skin or mucous membranes of the genitalia. Extragenital lesions are almost invariably associated with a large regional lymphadenopathy (bubos).

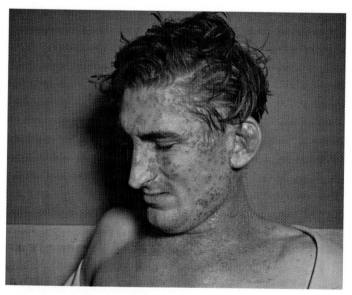

Figure 4–14.   Kaposi's varicelliform eruption

A serious complication of atopic dermatitis produced by the virus of herpes simplex or cowpox (vaccinia). The systemic reaction—fever, chills, lymphadenopathy—in this patient was severe.

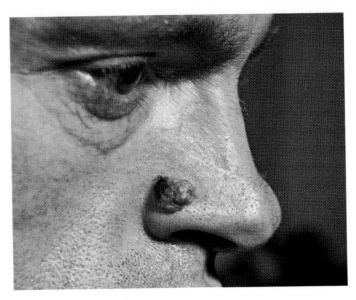

Figure 4–15. Herpes zoster (shingles)

Affecting the first branch of the trigeminal nerve. A most important type because of the possibility that the eye might become involved. This patient later developed invasive carcinoma of the mouth.

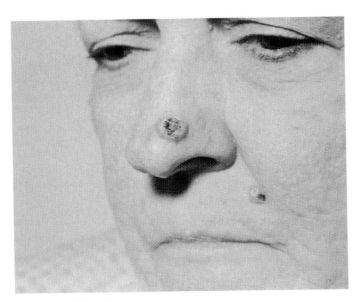

Figure 4–16. Lupus erythematosus

Searching study for systemic disease indicated. This patient proved well, aside from the extensive discoid lesions distributed principally to light-exposed sites.

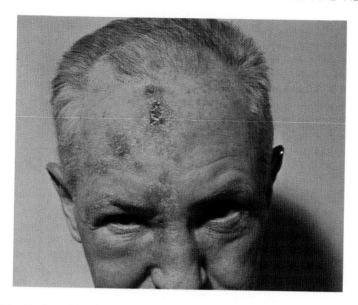

Figure 4–17.   Neglected basal cell epitheliomas of nasal fold and lower eyelid

Both lesions present rather difficult surgical or radiotherapeutic problems. The possibility of deeper extension of the tumor is significant. If the tumor had been recognized early, surgical removal would have been a simple matter.

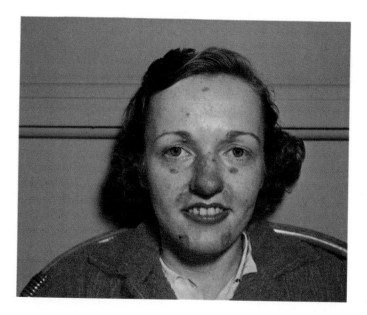

Figure 4–18.   Keratoacanthomas

A relatively benign, squamous cell-type tumor. Slow spontaneous involution usually occurs. Conservative removal indicated.

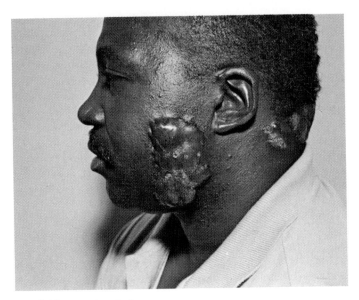

Figure 4–19. Keloids secondary to burn

Intralesional triamcinolone therapy is the treatment of choice, and the earlier it is started, the better.

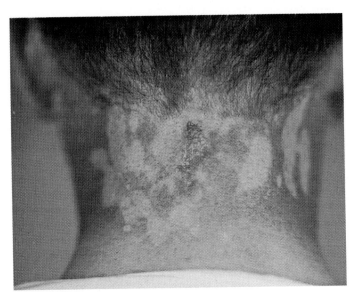

Figure 4–20. Factitial (self-produced) inflammation and scarring

The patient denied any manipulation. Such individuals may be seriously ill psychiatrically, but psychiatric management is usually unsuccessful.

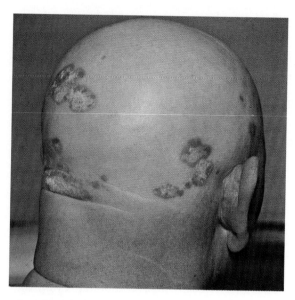

Figure 4–21.   Alopecia and psoriasis

An interesting but unusual combination of (1) alopecia areata, in this instance affecting the scalp totally and (2) typical lesions of psoriasis.

5

Dermatoses Affecting the Hands and Forearms

The hands and forearms are exposed to a wide variety of contactants, irritants, infectious agents and physical insults. It is not surprising, therefore, that a considerable number of dermatoses involve the hands and may remain localized there through their course. A lesion that would be relatively inconsequential elsewhere may produce varying degrees of disability, e.g., an irritated wart, an eczematous eruption, fissuring from psoriasis or ichthyosis.

An understanding of the following factors is helpful in dealing with hand eruptions.

1. The hands are subject to contact with a great variety of compounds that may have irritating or sensitizing effects. An inflammation that starts from one cause may be perpetuated by unrelated environmental irritants.

2. The hands are also subject to a variety of physical traumas, such as mechanical irritation, thermal insults and sunlight. Psoriasis or keratosis palmaris of the hands is accentuated by repeated trauma. Photosensitivity reactions may be marked on the backs of the hands.

3. Nonvenereal "primary inoculation syndromes" begin more frequently on the hands than on any part of the body. These range from common streptococcal and staphylococcic infections to less common conditions such as sporotrichosis and erysipeloid.

4. Any pruritic eruption tends to be particularly uncomfortable on the hands, especially the palms; the nerve endings are numerous and sensitive.

5. Sweating of the hands may be influenced by psychic factors. The amount of sweating may be astonishing under stress and is a significant factor in prolonging eczematous eruptions or chronic infection.

6. Involvement of the fingernails and surrounding soft tissues may present special problems in diagnosis and treatment. Such lesions, however, are rarely disabling, except in acute paronychial infection and cellulitis.

7. The hands are the most common sites of warts.

Diagnostic considerations in dermatosis affecting the hands and forearms are listed here. In this listing, somewhat in order of probability, the hands and forearms may be the only sites involved, but often, related lesions may be present elsewhere. In chronic inflammatory dermatosis of the hands, complete examination of the skin is highly advisable.

COMMON

Contact dermatitis (especially interdigital spaces and back of hands)
Warts
Neurodermatitis
Atopic dermatitis
Pompholyx
Superficial bacterial infections
Paronychial inflammation (traumatic, yeast and bacterial)
Fungal and yeast infections
Early syphilis (palms)

Scabies (palms and interdigital)
Psoriasis (papulosquamous) (especially nails and palms)
Vitiligo
Erythema multiforme
Ganglion
Ichthyosis
Photogenic reactions (especially backs of hands)
Actinic keratoses
Epithelioma

UNCOMMON

Radiodermatitis
Pustular psoriasis
Dermatitis repens
Raynaud's phenomenon and acrosclerosis
Primary inoculation syndromes (bacterial, fungal)
Variola
Systemic lupus erythematosus

Arsenical keratoses
Synovial cysts
Melanoma
Epidermolysis bullosa
Calcinosis
Xanthoma
Granuloma annulare
Keratosis palmaris

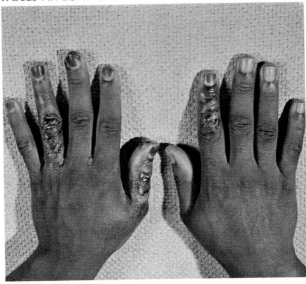

Figure 5–1.   Contact dermatitis due to Merthiolate

This patient had three episodes of inflammation following application of this compound for various reasons. Although the sensitization capacity of mercurial solutions is relatively low, there is little justification for their use because of their dubious value as operative preps or as treatment.

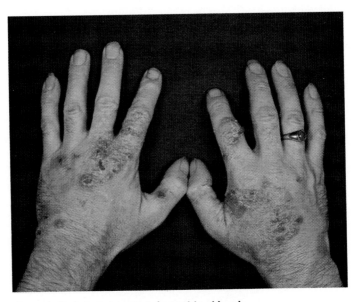

Figure 5–2.   Secondarily infected contact dermatitis of hands

Basic inflammation was related to frequent immersion in detergent solutions. This patient also was a food handler and therefore a prime public health menace.

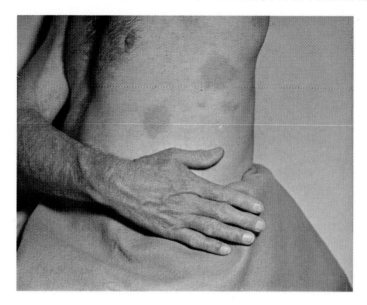

Figure 5–3.   Dermatitis of hands of physician due to procaine hydrochloride (Novocain)

The sites of inflammation on the trunk are from patch tests with various "caine" compounds, except for lidocaine which is chemically unrelated. This patient's sensitivity was so severe that he was forced to abandon his career in anesthesiology.

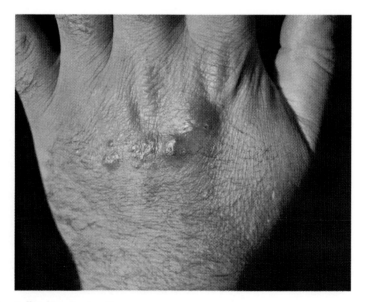

Figure 5–4.   Folliculitis due to oil

The incidence of such eruptions in mechanics is fairly high. Thorough cleansing after each work session is essential to control the condition. In some cases other secondary factors may make the inflammation self-perpetuating.

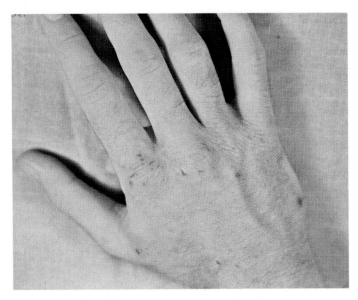

Figure 5–5.   Late atopic dermatitis

The hands are a common site of "neurodermatitis" in which the inflammation is perpetuated by a scratch-itch-scratch cycle. The scratching may be done quite unconsciously. Such areas are vulnerable to irritation or sensitization by occupational or therapeutic contactants.

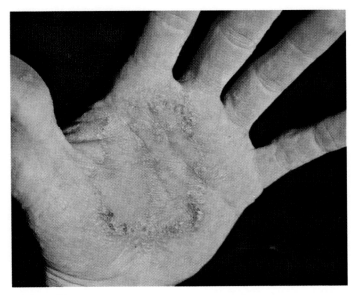

Figure 5–6.   Dermatitis repens

Dermatitis repens is an uncommon type of eczematoid eruption of the hands in which extension occurs with a circular continuous vesicular border. Bacterial infection plays a role, but other factors are also operative. It is usually very resistant to treatment.

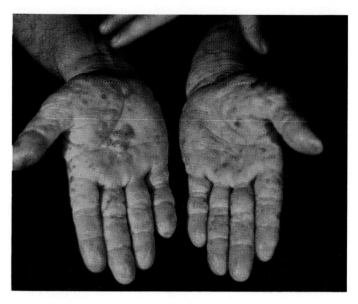

Figure 5–7. Dermatophytid

Dermatophytid is an inflammatory eruption, usually vesicular at the onset, occurring in association with a focus of fungal infection elsewhere on the skin, usually the feet. No fungi are demonstrable in the "id" lesion. There is an associated marked sensitivity to fungal antigens of the dermatophytic group.

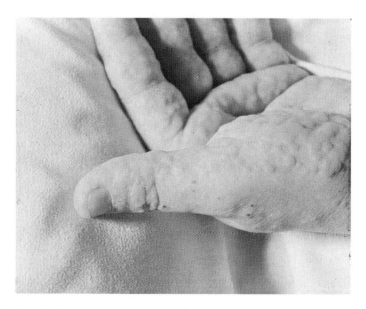

Figure 5–8. Pompholyx

Pompholyx is a vesicular eruption, characteristically seen on the hands. Attacks tend to occur in warm weather or after hyperhidrosis associated with nervous tension. This is not a variant of miliaria; the fluid in the vesicles is not sweat. Milder forms are very common. There is little or no inflammatory reaction at the onset.

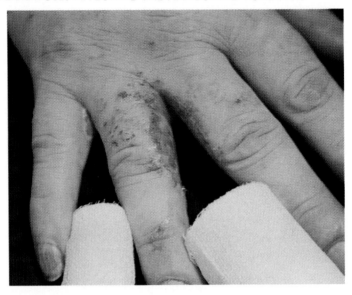

Figure 5–9.   Candidiasis (Moniliasis)

Intertriginous monilial (Candida) infection is seen most commonly in persons whose hands are subjected to frequent immersion in water. It may be part of a monilial overgrowth associated with broad spectrum antibiotic therapy. In females there may be an associated vaginal infection.

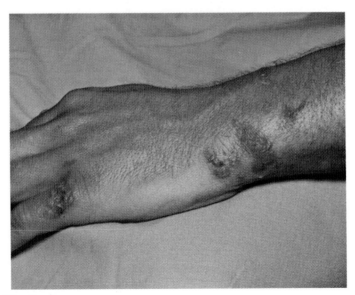

Figure 5–10.   Pyoderma

Mixed infection by coagulase-positive staphylococci and beta-hemolytic streptococci. Systemic antibiotic therapy is essential to adequate management.

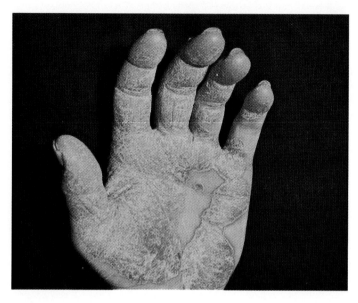

Figure 5–11.   Psoriasis

Psoriasis may sometimes be largely restricted to the palms. The picture is similar to that on the soles. Sterile pustules may be present (pustular psoriasis). Lesions are most marked on areas of pressure, and painful fissuring may occur, especially in cold weather or after trauma.

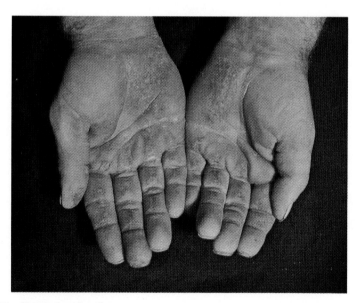

Figure 5–12.   Keratosis palmaris

As in the case with inherited keratosis of the soles, keratosis palmaris may become aggravated by trauma. Not much can be done except to provide protection with gloves and to use keratolytic and emollient agents.

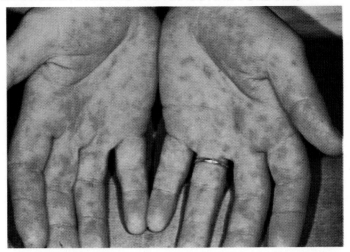

Figure 5–13. Characteristic secondary syphilis of the palms

This is an almost pathognomonic clinical picture. If the lesions tend to be pustular, however, together with a systemic reaction, consideration must be given to smallpox or varioloid.

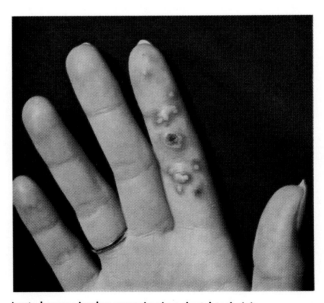

Figure 5–14. Acute herpes simplex occurring in a dental technician

This inoculation complex is not uncommon in dental practice. If it is a primary infection (unusual in adults), the associated lymphadenopathy and systemic reaction may be severe. (Courtesy of Dr. G. W. Hambrick, Jr.)

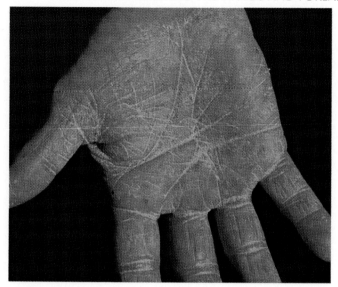

Figure 5–15.   Chronic *Trichophyton rubrum* infection of palms, a very characteristic clinical picture

Only one hand may be involved. This infection was almost never cured prior to availability of griseofulvin, prolonged courses of which are necessary.

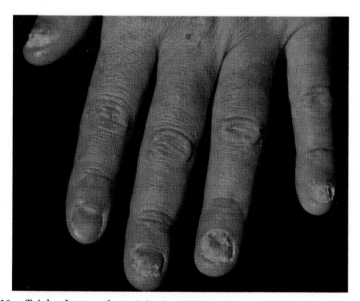

Figure 5–16.   *Trichophyton rubrum* infection of fingernails

It is often difficult to differentiate this condition from psoriasis or nail dystrophy following chronic dermatitis of the surrounding skin.

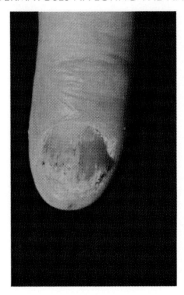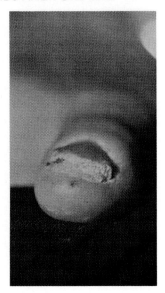

Figure 5–17.   Psoriasis of nails

This may be the only evidence of the disease at times, particularly in children. Usually there is some involvement of toenails as well. There may be episodes of relatively low-grade paronychial inflammation. Very unresponsive to treatment.

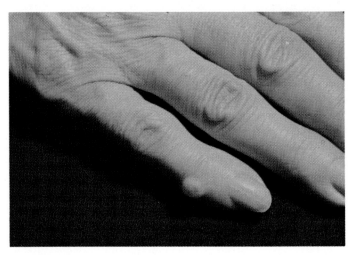

Figure 5–18.   Synovial cyst

A banal lesion, sometimes moderately painful. Often associated with some arthritic changes of the distal phalanges. Responsive to injection of triamcinolone into cyst in most cases. Surgical repair is rarely necessary.

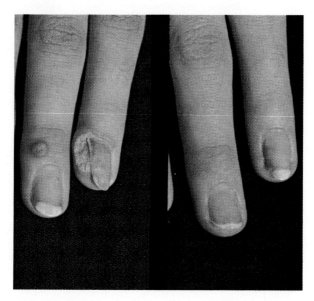

Figure 5–19. Warts (verrucae), before and after chemotherapy with nitric-acid-phenol-salicylic acid plaster

The hands are the most common site of warts. All treatments are illogical in the absence of any specific antiviral agent. Application of liquid nitrogen is a useful treatment. Paronychial warts sometimes prove incurable. (Courtesy of Dr. G. W. Hambrick, Jr.)

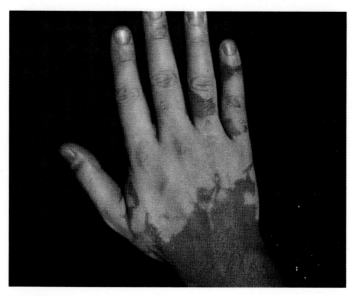

Figure 5–20. Vitiligo

Vitiligo may appear anywhere on the skin, but lesions on exposed surfaces are the more important for cosmetic reasons and because of increased vulnerability to sunlight. There is no satisfactory treatment. There may be an associated anemia.

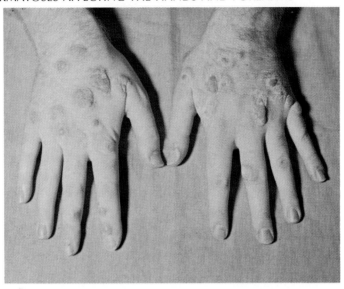

Figure 5–21.   Erythema multiforme

The "target" lesions of erythema multiforme are highly characteristic. Lesions are usually found elsewhere and may vary in type (multiform) from urticarial to purpuric to bullous. The type in which there is involvement of the mouth, conjunctiva and urethra is the most severe and may be fatal.

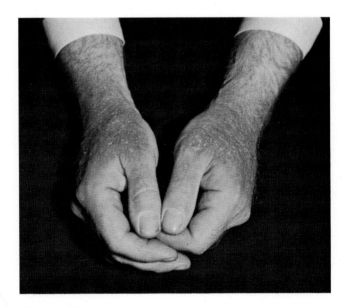

Figure 5–22.   Photosensitivity

Photosensitivity reactions are on the increase. Many drugs, in this instance demethylchlortet-racycline, are capable of inducing sensitivity to sunlight. Contact photosensitivity to topical agents must also be considered.

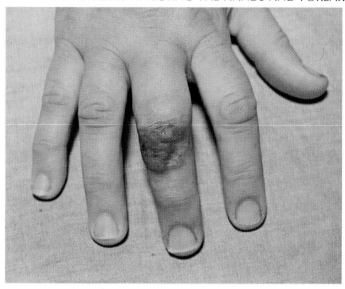

Figure 5–23.   Anthrax

Anthrax is primarily a disease of sheep, horses and cattle and is a risk to persons who come into contact with the hides of these animals. It is one of the most explosive of the primary inoculation syndromes of the skin. Its prepenicillin mortality was from 5 to 10 per cent.

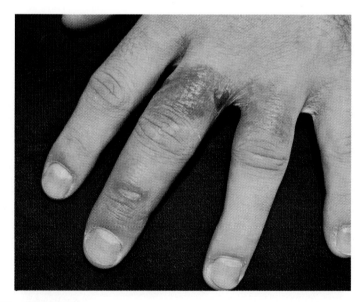

Figure 5–24.   Erysipeloid

Erysipeloid is another example of a very acute occupational infection seen in persons who handle fish and shellfish and, occasionally, meat or poultry. The systemic manifestations are distinctly less than those of anthrax. The history is usually obvious and clearcut. The causative organism is *Erysipelothrix rhusiopathiae*.

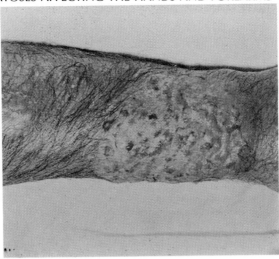

Figure 5–25.   Tinea profunda

Ringworm infections acquired from animals tend to be more inflammatory than those from human sources. In this infection, acquired from a cow, the causative organism was *Trichophyton mentagrophytes*. The systemic reaction was almost nil, and spontaneous healing occurred eventually.

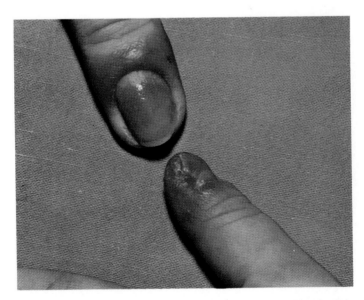

Figure 5–26.   Paronychial inflammation in husband and wife, caused by Candida (Monilia)

Conjugal genital candidiasis is also not uncommon.

6

Dermatoses Affecting the Trunk, Axillae, and Anogenital Region

TRUNK AND AXILLAE

The skin of the trunk, the largest body surface, may be the site of almost any disease affecting the skin. Relatively few diseases are confined to this region, however, in contrast with areas such as the hands, the feet and the genitalia. Most of the common diseases affecting the skin of the trunk and axillae may be recognized promptly on close inspection. Much can be accomplished diagnostically if the more common syndromes are either tentatively confirmed or ruled out.

These diseases are as follows:

COMMON

Acne—grades III and IV (acne conglobata)
Seborrheic dermatitis (presternal and interscapular areas
Tinea versicolor
Pityriasis rosea
Psoriasis
Tinea corporis (especially in tropical climates or in immunosuppressed patients)
Secondary syphilis
Infections, bacterial
Miliaria

Contact dermatitis
Atopic dermatitis
Nummular dermatitis
Urticaria
Seborrheic keratoses
Herpes zoster
Rubella
Rubeola
Varicella
Pediculosis corporis
Scabies
Cherry (senile) angiomas

UNCOMMON

Bathing suit hairy nevus
Bowen's disease (epithelioma in situ)
Erythema perstans
Macula caeruleae (with pediculosis)

Mastocytosis (urticaria pigmentosa)
Mycosis fungoides
Paget's disease (female breast areola)

Acne.   Acne becomes more than a cosmetic problem when it involves the trunk rather than just the face, and it may produce considerable disability in the form of numerous inflamed, tender cystic lesions. The most marked lesions are often on the shoulders and upper back and may make pack carrying or the wearing of football gear impossible. In its most severe form, it may involve the posterior scalp, the axillae and the inguinal regions. In the latter two areas the apocrine glands are infected. This condition is known as hidradenitis suppurativa and may be so persistent and severe as to require surgical excision and grafting.

Seborrheic Dermatitis.   The favorite site of this reddish scaling eruption is the presternal area. There is often some concomitant involvement of the scalp, the ears, the axillae or the crural folds. The dermatitis may become very extensive.

Tinea Versicolor.   This is a banal, harmless, superficial yeast infection that produces small round fawn-colored to brownish scaling patches without any inflammation. The lesions are usually distributed principally to the upper portion of the trunk. The affected areas do not tan as does normal skin, and this may produce a bizarre appearance.

Pityriasis Rosea.   This is a highly characteristic eruption that almost always affects the trunk. The initial lesion is a moderately inflamed annular patch with a characteristic narrow scaling border. A week or less after its appearance there is ordinarily a shower of similar lesions, usually smaller than the initial ones. The eruption is frequently misdiagnosed as ringworm. The primary plaque may not occur in some cases.

Psoriasis.   In extensive cases of this disease, the trunk is almost always involved. The lesions may be solid red scaling plaques or annular lesions, often with striking geometric patterns. The borders of the lesions are usually sharp, with an abrupt transition from affected to normal skin.

Tinea Corporis.   Ringworm affecting the trunk is not commonly seen in temperate climates. In subtropical or tropical environments, however, the infection may become very extensive and inflammatory on the trunk. The characteristic initial lesion is round and scaling, with varying degrees of inflammation of the border. In many instances, however, particularly in hot climates and under poor hygienic conditions, the characteristic annular pattern may disappear.

Secondary Syphilis.   The trunk is not as commonly involved in this infection as are the genitalia, mucous membranes, palms and soles. On the trunk, the lesions of early syphilis may vary from a faint, barely visible, roseola to very prominent papular or plaque-like lesions, particularly if the infection has gone undetected for many weeks or months.

Miliaria.   The trunk is the favorite site of involvement in "heat rash." If the blockage of the sweat ducts is very superficial, only clear, symptomless small vesicles are seen. If the blockage is deeper, however, the patient sweats *into* rather than *onto* his skin, and the itch stimulus

can be acute and severe. Obese persons and those with atopic or seborrheic dermatitis are particularly prone to miliaria.

Contact Dermatitis.   Although reactions to external contactants are
much less common on the trunk and in the axillae than on exposed
areas of the body, they do occur, and the cause is often missed. The
most frequent offenders are materials in underclothing, particularly
elastic components, nickel fasteners and various deodorants and other
cosmetics.

Text continued on page 98.

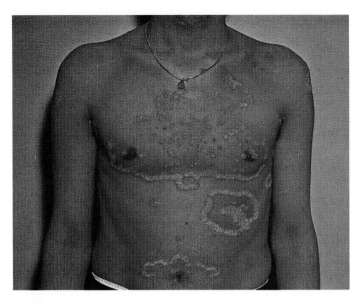

Figure 6–1. Psoriasis

This disease, in its most characteristic form, is among the easiest of all eruptions to diagnose. About 2 per cent of all white adults have it, though frequently in very mild form. In extensive involvement, psoriasis is a "socially very disabling" disease.

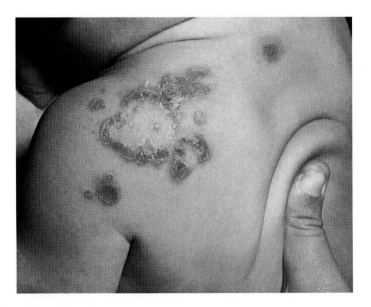

Figure 6–2. Bullous impetigo

This superficial infection, ordinarily caused initially by streptococci, involves the face most commonly but is frequently more extensive. Systemic antibiotic therapy is essential; dependence should not be placed on topical therapy alone.

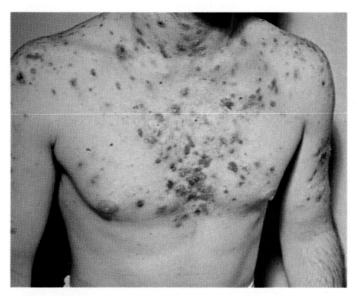

Figure 6–3.   Severe extensive acne of the chest

Explosive acne of this type is fairly common in a warm humid climate (tropical acne). The patient may have had little or no evidence of acne previously. Significant scarring is, unfortunately, inevitable. The psychic depression induced by this painful and disfiguring eruption is often severe. Hypertrophic scarring is common.

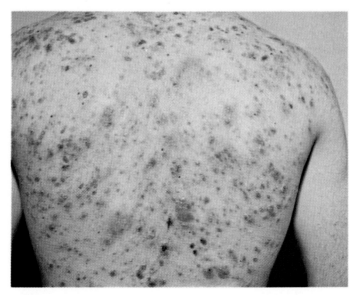

Figure 6–4.   Acne of the back

Lesions of this type are often painful and make the carrying of heavy gear or contact athletic activity impossible. The acne frequently cannot be brought under control until the patient is removed to a cooler climate. Prolonged antibiotic therapy is usually necessary.

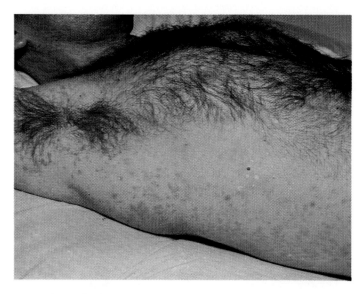

Figure 6–5. Measles (Rubeola)

In any suddenly appearing eruption accompanied by fever the possibility of an infectious exanthem must always be considered. In measles the principal signs and symptoms are (1) a prodrome of 4 days or longer—with fever, coryza, photophobia and cough, (2) Koplik spots in the mouth and (3) a morbilliform rash, with lethargy, headache and marked photophobia—persisting for 3 to 5 days.

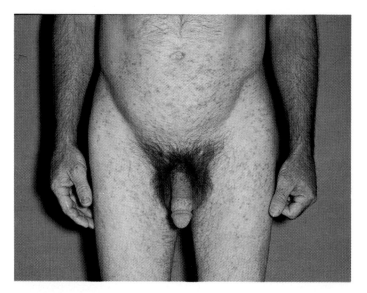

Figure 6–6. Pediculosis corporis

The "cooties" of World War I achieved much notoriety and caused considerable disability and secondary infection. DDT prevented this almost completely in World War II. Occasional cases may be seen, however, especially in individuals coming in close contact with native populations who practice poor hygiene or in prisoners of war. Unfortunately, DDT-containing dusting powder is almost unobtainable at present.

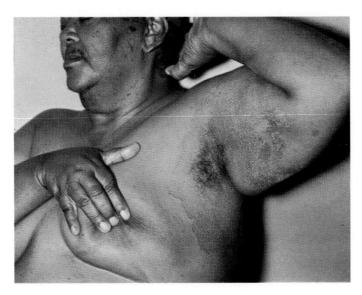

Figure 6–7. Erythrasma

This superficial bacterial infection is seen most commonly in warm climates and in obese patients. It resembles a ringworm infection but may be promptly differentiated by a coral red fluorescence when examined under a Wood's light.

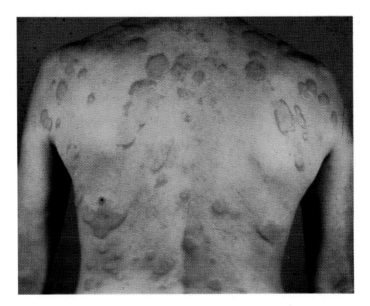

Figure 6–8. Chronic urticaria

Urticaria (hives) is a localized edema of the skin, usually accompanied by considerable itching. The affected area is white to pink, and the border is usually redder than the rest of the lesion. In an acute first attack of urticaria, a specific drug (most commonly penicillin) or a food can often be established as the cause. In chronic urticaria a specific cause is often impossible to establish, and many cases are not truly allergic in origin.

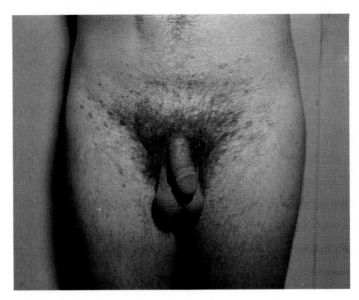

Figure 6–9. Pityriasis rosea

Typical ringed, moderately inflamed lesions with a scaling border. Duration 6 to 12 weeks. Treatment is often unnecessary, but if considered advisable, a short course of corticosteroid therapy is usually curative.

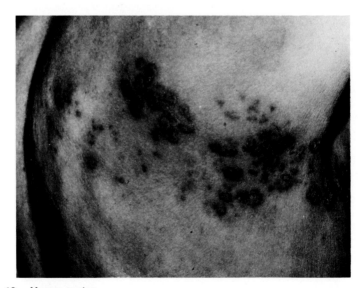

Figure 6–10. Herpes zoster

Typical tense grouped vesicles in a linear neural distribution. The pain varies, tending to be more severe in older persons. The causative virus (VZ) is the same as that producing varicella (chickenpox). Occasionally encountered in association with a lymphoma, particularly Hodgkin's disease. (Courtesy of G. W. Hambrick, Jr.)

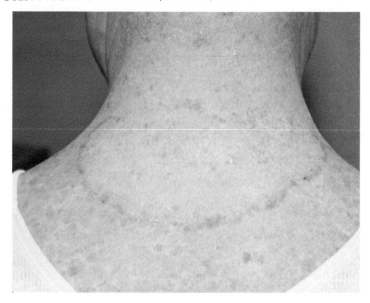

Figure 6–11. Tinea corporis

Typical ring-shaped lesions. Rapidly responsive to griseofulvin as a rule, except under adverse environmental and hygienic conditions or in persons with severe systemic disease, e.g., uncontrolled diabetes or lymphoma.

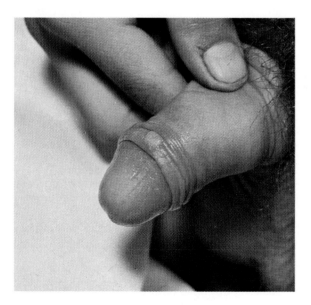

Figure 6–12. Chancre

The primary lesion of syphilis. This lesion appears two or more weeks after infectious sexual exposure. It is characteristically hard and painless and is associated with bilateral inguinal lymph node enlargement. Spirochetes are easily demonstrable by darkfield microscopy in serum obtained from such a lesion.

ANOGENITAL REGION

The genitalia, crural folds, perianal region, buttocks and upper inner thighs are common sites of a considerable number of rashes and ulcers. Inflammatory lesions of various types are frequently more pruritic or painful in this region than on most other parts of the skin surface. They are also aggravated by poor hygienic conditions, excessive weight and stresses of physical activity. These diseases are as follows:

COMMON DERMATOSES

Males	Females*
Fungal infections	Candidiasis
Candidiasis	Contact dermatitis
Circumscribed neurodermatitis	Warts
Contact dermatitis	Herpetic vulvovaginitis (adult)
Seborrheic dermatitis	Early syphilis
Erythrasma	Erythrasma
Warts	Intertrigo of undetermined cause
Herpes simplex types I and II	Parasitic infestations
Early syphilis	Scabies
Parasitic infestations	Lice
Scabies	Trichomonad
Lice	Pinworms
Trichomoniasis	Creeping eruption
Pinworms	Nevi
Creeping eruption	Epidermal cysts
Chancroid	Mucous cysts
Psoriasis	Acrochordon
	Traumatic hematoma

UNCOMMON DERMATOSES

Males	Females*
Lichen planus	Herpetic vulvovaginitis (children)
Granuloma inguinale	Hidradenoma
Lymphogranuloma venereum	Mesonephric duct cysts
Molluscum contagiosum	Fox-Fordyce disease
Carcinoma-in-situ (Bowen's disease)	Bartholin cysts
Paget's disease	Varicosities
Behcet's disease	Drug eruptions
Lichen sclerosus et atrophicus	
Leukoplakia	
Squamous cell carcinoma	
Hidradenitis suppurativa	
Drug eruptions	

*Adapted from Friedrich, E. G., Jr.: Vulvar Disease. Philadelphia, W. B. Saunders Co., 1976.

Venereal Ulcerative Lesions — Chancre and Chancroid. The primary lesion of syphilis is usually a hard painless lesion associated with a nonfluctuant lymphadenopathy, the bubo. Chancroid, by contrast, produces a more imflammatory ulcer that tends to increase in size and is associated with a fluctuant bubo that may be quite painful. The ulcers of chancroid are frequently multiple, in contrast to the single chancre of syphilis. Lesions of secondary syphilis frequently involve the genitalia, both in males and in females.

Fungal Infection. This most commonly involves the upper inner thighs but may be much more extensive, particularly in tropical environments. The lesions are usually ring shaped, hence the term ringworm.

Moniliasis (Candidiasis, "Yeast Infection"). The most commonly affected areas are the crural folds, gluteal cleft and perianal region. In its chronic phase in intertriginous areas, the infection appears as sodden, white macerated skin with a moderately inflamed border. Acute flare-ups are characterized by increased redness and extension of the inflammation in the form of small superficial pustules. Intramarital "ping-pong" relapses may be seen. In persistent or severe infections, the possibility of diabetes must be considered.

Erythrasma. This superficial bacterial infection is characterized by brownish scaling patches, ordinarily with relatively little inflammation.

Herpes Simplex ("Cold Sore"). The lesion may appear recurrently on the genitalia. This is usually Type II of HVH (herpes virus hominis). In the female, HVH Type II infections may play a significant role in the development of cancer of the cervix.

Psoriasis. In chronic form, this eruption shows the characteristic, sharply outlined, dull red scaling patches. If the lesions are in folds, they become whitish and macerated and may resemble a yeast infection; indeed, the two diseases may coexist.

Lichen Planus. This characteristic eruption may be confined to the glans penis.

Seborrheic Dermatitis. In extensive form, this commonly involves the folds of the anogenital region. There will almost always be concurrent involvement of the scalp, axillae and other areas.

Contact Dermatitis. Although the anogenital region is not as common a site for reactions to external irritants and sensitizers as are exposed areas of the skin, such reactions do occur there. In poison ivy dermatitis, the noxious antigen is frequently transferred to the genitalia by the hands.

"Scratch" Dermatitis (Localized Neurodermatitis). The genitalia and perianal region are erogenous zones that are very "itchy." Once pruritus occurs there, whatever the original cause, it tends to be perpetuated by scratching and can sometimes last for many years. This results in thickening and darkening of the skin. The relation of increased itching to stress is often clear-cut; some persons scratch instead of biting their nails or smoking more cigarettes.

Pediculosis.   The "crabs" of this type of louse infection are easily visible if looked for. Itching is usually marked, and there may be secondary bacterial infection. Sometimes only nits are visible.

Scabies ("Seven Year Itch").   The small burrowing mite *Sarcoptes scabiei* is less commonly encountered in the skin of man today. Under conditions of dislocation of the civilian population, however, as in the blitz in Britain in World War II, it may become endemic. Pruritic papules on the penis should *always* arouse suspicion of scabies. The infestation may be endemic and very severe in residents of institutions for the mentally retarded.

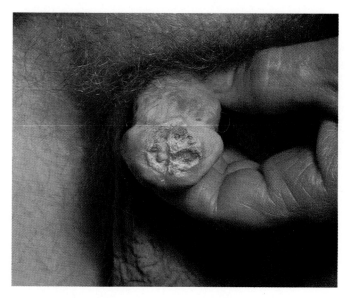

Figure 6–13.   Squamous cell cancer of the glans penis

Such a lesion is almost always preceded by a longstanding "precancerous" condition.

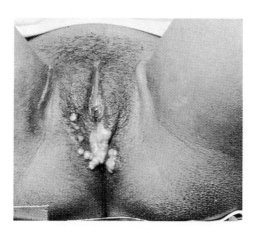

Figure 6–14.   Condylomata of secondary syphilis

These lesions, which may be mistaken for "venereal" warts, appear several weeks to months after the initial infection. They swarm with spirochetes. Unprotected sexual contact of a non-syphilitic individual with a patient of this type carries virtually a 100 per cent risk of infection.

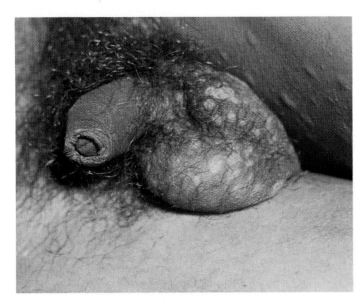

Figure 6–15. Papular lesions of secondary syphilis on the scrotum

Note lesions on inner thigh as well. This patient has a spirochetemia, i.e., organisms of syphilis circulating in the blood stream and lodging in the skin and various internal organs.

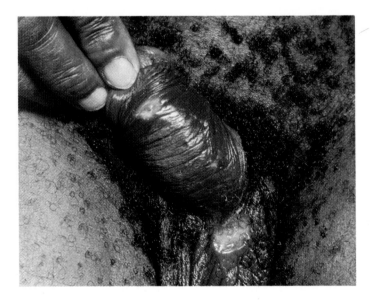

Figure 6–16. Chancroid

These lesions tend to appear sooner after sexual exposure than does syphilis. Multiple lesions are common. The ulcers are often painful and usually soft. The associated bubo is usually fluctuant and may drain. It should not be incised, but rather drained through a large bore needle. It may coexist with syphilis.

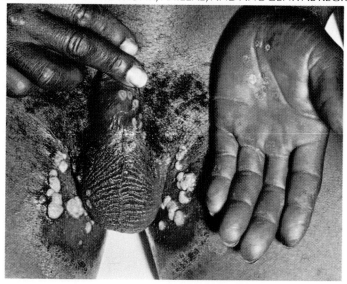

Figure 6–17.   Another example of widespread lesions of secondary syphilis

The palmar lesions are very characteristic, and a diagnosis of syphilis should receive first consideration in dry papular lesions of this area. This patient is a public health menace of the first order.

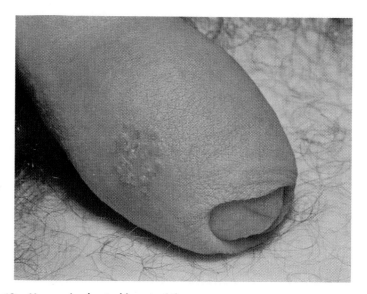

Figure 6–18.   Herpes simplex (cold sore) of the prepuce

Such lesions may occur repeatedly at or near the same site. They are usually caused by herpes simplex virus acrotype II.

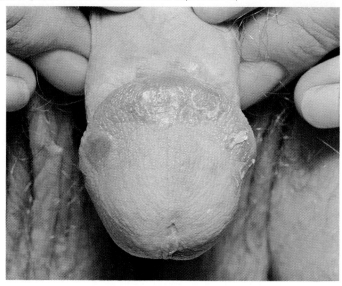

Figure 6–19.   Psoriasis

Dry scaling lesions of the glans penis. Ordinarily accompanied by lesions elsewhere, especially the scalp, elbows and knees.

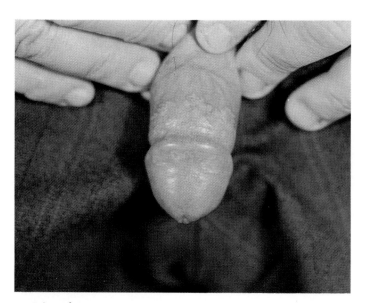

Figure 6–20.   Lichen planus

A very characteristic though uncommon chronic eruption of the penis. Usually associated with lesions elsewhere, especially the mucous membranes of the mouth.

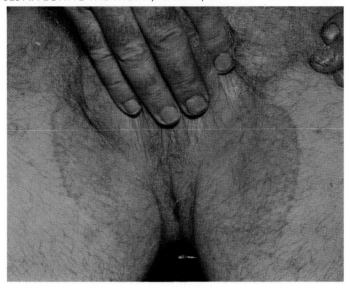

Figure 6–21.   Tinea cruris (jock itch)

Characteristic annular, scaling, inflamed lesions of the upper thighs and scrotum. Fungi are easily demonstrable in scales scraped from the lesions. Griseofulvin therapy is ordinarily very effective, but several new topically applied compounds have become available.

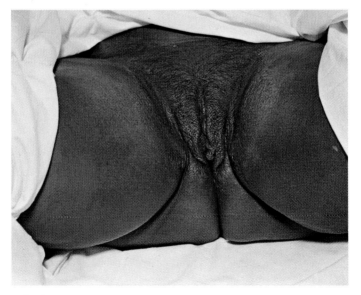

Figure 6–22.   Erythrasma

A superficial bacterial infection. Most common in obese persons living in a hot climate. The affected areas show a coral red fluorescence when examined with a Wood's light.

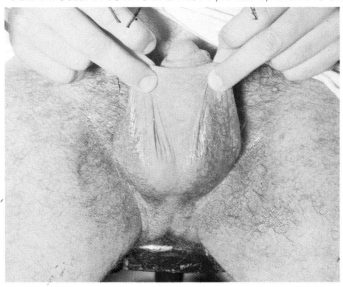

Figure 6–23. Intertrigo

Disabling inflammation of apposing skin surfaces in the genital area. No specific microorganism was demonstrably responsible. The eruption is due to a combination of heat, sweating, friction and poor hygiene.

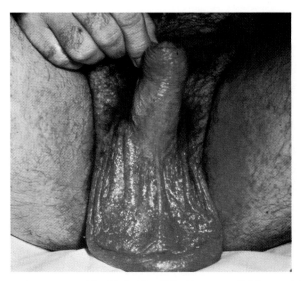

Figure 6–24. Severe acute Moniliasis (Candidiasis), a superficial yeast infection

There is evidence of overtreatment, to which the scrotum is particularly susceptible.

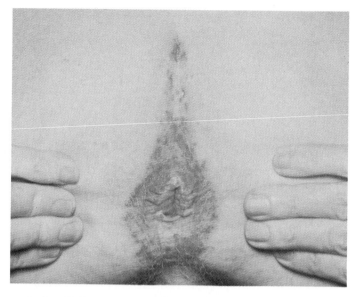

Figure 6–25.   Perianal inflammation caused by Monilia

Similar changes may be associated with psoriasis and seborrheic dermatitis. Itching may be extreme, and the inflammation perpetuated by scratching.

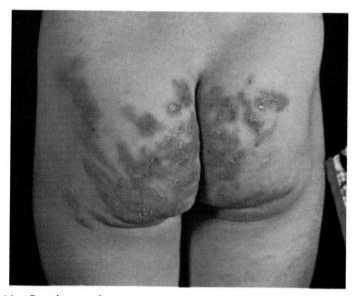

Figure 6–26.   Creeping eruption

A burrowing irregularly linear inflammation produced by the larva of dog or cat hookworm. The infestation is acquired by contact with moist soil or sand which has been contaminated by dog or cat feces.

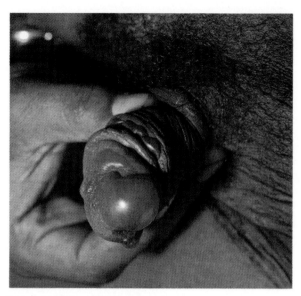

Figure 6–27.   Bullous dermatitis medicamentosa

The patient was extremely sensitive to medications containing iodine. The eruption developed full blown within 24 hours of ingestion.

7

Dermatoses Affecting the Feet and Lower Legs

The feet and lower legs are a very common site of a considerable variety of minor to disabling dermatoses, as abundantly attested to by the continued growth of the specialty of podiatric medicine. Erect posture, with the resultant continued stress upon the muscles, bones, joints and vasculature of the lower extremities, plays an important part in determining the type and distribution of diseases seen on the feet and lower legs. Some of the specific factors leading to diseases of the skin and subcutaneous system are as follows:

1. The wearing of heavy, occlusive footgear, as in the case of foot soldiers, with inadequte aeration, accumulation of sweat and maldistribution of skin pressures and orthopedic support.

2. With many types of footgear, an opportunity for overgrowth of a wide variety of fungi and bacteria.

3. The sensitizing effects of several shoe components, adhesives, dyes, synthetic leathers and other materials.

4. The induction of latent disease by friction, e.g., psoriasis and epidermolysis bullosa.

5. Responses to stressful environmental factors of temperature and moisture, e.g., the trench foot of World War II and the "paddie foot" of Vietnam, both capable of inducing prolonged disability.

6. Susceptibility to viral infection with warts, highly transmissible in family bathrooms and gymnasiums.

7. Excessive sweating, often in response to psychic stress.

8. Anatomic variation, as in persons whose toe interspaces are occluded and do not spread when the individual stands.

9. Lack of scrupulous hygiene in many individuals, particularly with respect to rinsing and drying between the toes.

10. Vulnerability of the skin in persons with underlying vascular disease, e.g., stasis, diabetes and arterial occlusion.

The following are diagnostic considerations in foot and lower leg dermatoses.

COMMON

Superficial fungal and yeast
  infections
Stasis dermatitis
Warts
Callosities
Superficial and deep bacterial
  infections
Contact dermatitis
Atopic dermatitis

Drug eruption
Insect bites
Ichthyosis and keratosis plantaris
Purpuric and hemosiderin
  pigmentation
Larva migrans (creeping eruption)
Corns
Vasculitis
Psoriasis

UNCOMMON

Lichen amyloidosis
Chromoblastomycosis
Pretibial myxedema
Diabetic dermopathy
Necrobiosis diabeticorum
Elephantiasis nostras
Epidermolysis bullosa
Erythema induratum
Mycetoma
Swimming pool granuloma

Bromoderma
Mal perforans
Sickle cell anemia
Tumors of various types, especially
  melanoma and Kaposi's
  hemorrhagic sarcoma
Keratoderma blennorrhagica
Erythema nodosum
Lichen planus

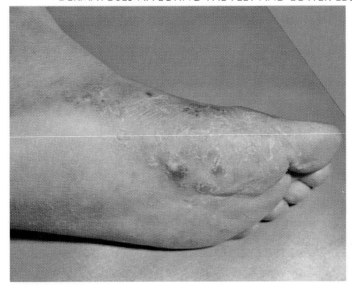

Figure 7–1. Acute fungal infection due to *Trichophyton mentagrophytes*

Flare-ups occur from a warm environment, continuous wearing of occlusive footgear and chronic immersion. Highly susceptible to secondary bacterial infection, beginning in this case. May be accompanied by allergic dermatophytid eruption of hands.

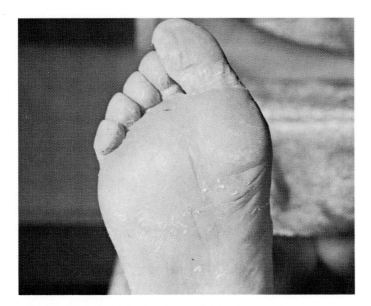

Figure 7–2. Chronic dry fungal infection due to *Trichophyton rubrum*

Uncomfortable at times, but rarely disabling. Not infrequently, only one foot is involved. A typical distribution is in those areas which might be covered by a moccasin.

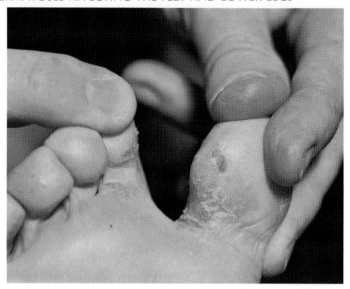

Figure 7–3. Typical interdigital fungal infection

Usually responsive to good foot hygiene and topical and systemic antifungal agents. Local corticosteroid therapy also effective temporarily, but may favor the growth of fungi. Confirmation of the diagnosis by scrapings is very desirable; other conditions may produce this picture.

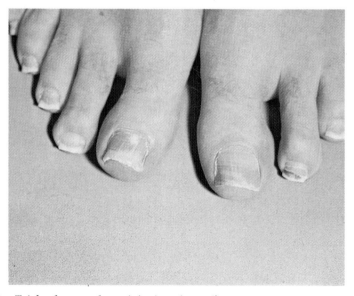

Figure 7–4. *Trichophyton rubrum* infection of toenails

Incurable, even after many months of griseofulvin therapy. Attempt to cure usually futile except to control inflammatory flare-ups on skin.

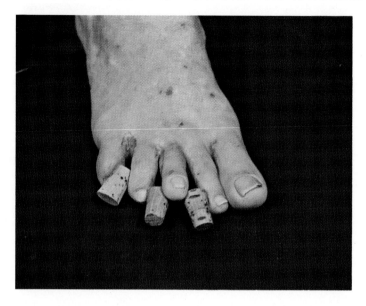

Figure 7–5. Streptococcal secondary infection of chronic intertriginous inflammation

Systemic antibiotic therapy indicated, preferably penicillin or erythromycin. Dependence should not be placed on topical therapy alone.

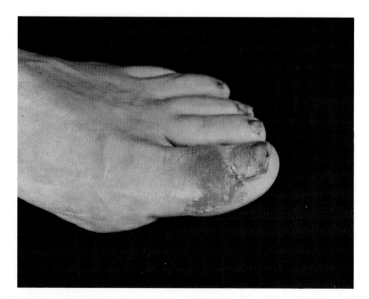

Figure 7–6. Contact dermatitis with early secondary infection

Should be treated on a nonambulatory basis until infection is under control. If underlying dermatitis is due to component of footgear, frequent relapses and chronicity are the rule. The stain of the nails from $KMnO_4$ foot soaks.

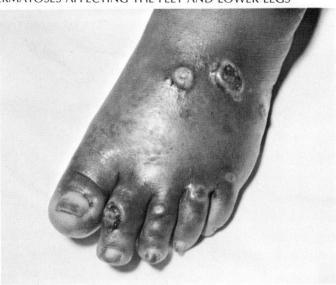

Figure 7–7.   Multiple ecthymatous ulcers at sites of trauma from footgear

Staphylococci commonly produce these deep ulcerations. A mixed flora may, however, be present, making culture and antibiotic sensitivity tests advisable. Recurrent lesions and extension of the infection are common in patients with diabetes, peripheral vascular disease and immune suppression. Occlusion, heat and moisture may also produce relapse. Therapy usually requires bed rest and specific systemic antibiotic therapy.

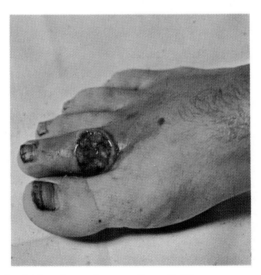

Figure 7–8.   Rapidly developing ulcer and surrounding cellulitis

May develop very rapidly under adverse climatic and hygienic conditions. Searching bacteriologic study indicated. Sometimes termed "tropical ulcer."

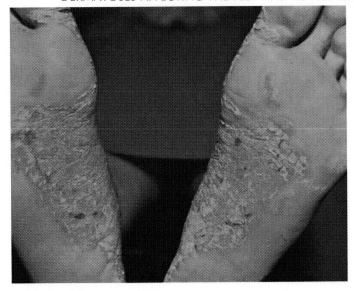

Figure 7–9. Psoriasis of soles

Sharply marginated plaques. Disabling fissures are common. Often very resistant to treatment. Crops of pustules may be noted.

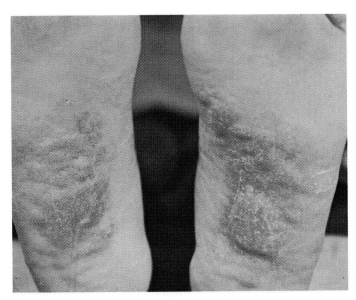

Figure 7–10.   Contact dermatitis of soles due to sensitivity to rubber sole insert

Dermatitis developed for first time after prolonged immersion.

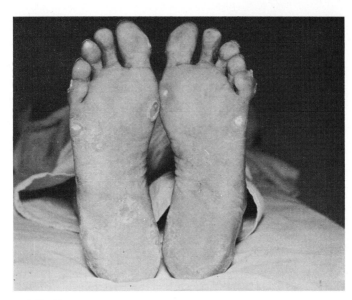

Figure 7–11.   Callosities

Partially controllable by prevention of trauma and removal of excessive keratin by paring down or applying salicylic acid compounds. The topical application of 10 to 40 per cent urea in an oily lotion may be helpful.

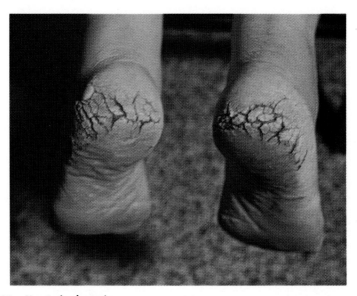

Figure 7–12.   Keratosis plantaris

A congenitally endowed abnormal response to pressure and trauma. May become markedly accentuated under conditions of heavy labor or military duty. Note the fibroma which has developed on the left heel.

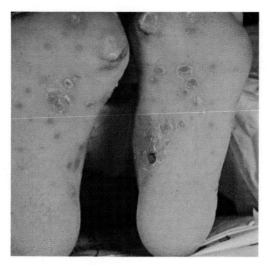

Figure 7–13.   Papular secondary syphilis

An almost pathognomonic eruption. Palms are usually involved as well, plus variable lesions elsewhere. Such lesions may become temporarily more marked following penicillin therapy (Herxheimer reaction).

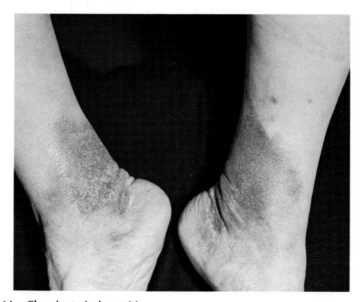

Figure 7–14.   Chronic stasis dermatitis

The involved areas are particularly prone to sensitization from applied medication. Relapses are common.

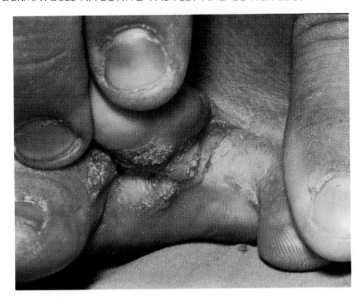

Figure 7–19.   Warts between toes

Warts in any moist macerated area are white and tend to become enlarged. The conditions are so suitable for the growth of the virus that cure is often difficult.

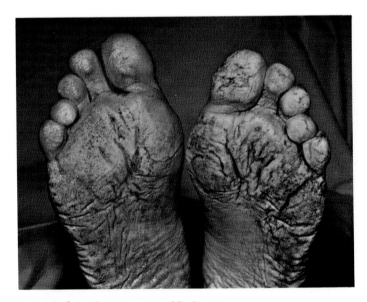

Figure 7–20.   Tropical wet foot injury ("paddie foot")

Due to prolonged immersion in warm tropical waters. The thick macerated stratum corneum is cast off, and the feet are intolerant of trauma for some time. A source of much disability in Vietnam.

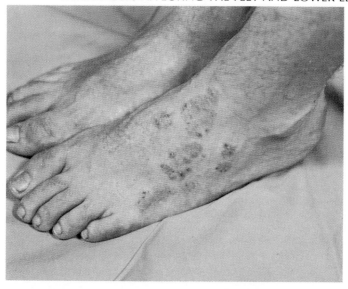

Figure 7–21.   Fungal infection at site of abrasion from rough sock

Any type of superficial injury to the skin, whether mechanical or through maceration, favors invasion and growth of fungi.

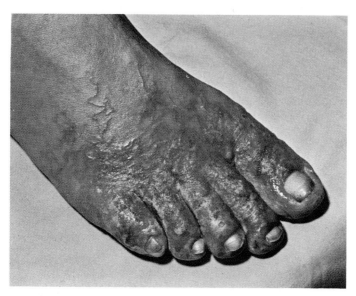

Figure 7–22.   Larva migrans (creeping eruption)

Burrows and inflammation produced by the larvae of cat or dog hookworm. Acquired by contact with fecally contaminated sand or soil. Lesions largely obscured by overtreatment in this patient.

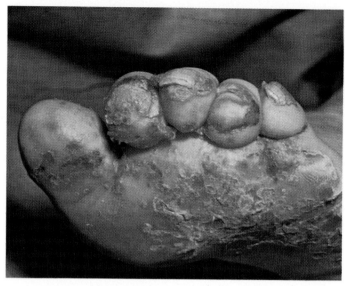

Figure 7–23.   Keratoderma blennorrhagica

An uncommon but highly distinctive psoriasiform eruption which may occur in Reiter's disease (nonspecific urethritis, arthritis, conjunctivitis and balanitis). Probably bacterial in origin, but responsible organism not yet established with certainty.

Acne, Rosacea and Miliaria | 8

ACNE

Acne is a disease so common as to be almost a normal physiologic response to adolescence, though the precise incidence in children of various ethnic groups, dietary customs and climatic environments has not been determined exactly. All that can be said is that it is frequently encountered and that it varies in severity from minor cosmetic changes that pass spontaneously with little or no residue to an ugly, often painful, disabling, scarring inflammatory process that may remain troublesome far into adult life and have serious psychic implications.*

The Course of Acne

In the prognosis and treatment of acne, it is necessary to have some knowledge of the etiologic factors influencing it and of its various clinical forms. The latter are so variable as to make it difficult to cover them with the umbrella of a single disease designation. Many factors have varying influences, and the early and late morphologic changes differ widely.

Infantile Acne. In the skin of the newborn infant, the sebaceous glands are small and relatively inactive, although occasionally stimulated by maternal androgens, with a resultant scattering of open and closed comedones. These comedones are evanescent and of no importance. The clinical picture may sometimes be simulated by overzealous application of comedogenic baby oils.

Pubertal Acne. Under the influence of increasing androgenic serum levels at puberty both in boys and in girls, the sebaceous gland (see Fig.1–11) enlarges and secretes increasing amounts of sebum by casting off oil-bearing cells mixed with keratin. This mixture soon becomes heavily colonized with *Propionibacterium acnes.*

---

*See the magnum opus, Plewig, G., and Kligman, A. M.: Acne: Morphogenesis and Treatment. Springer-Verlag, New York, 1975. This profusely illustrated monograph is highly recommended to any physician wishing to delve into modern concepts of acne. Various papers by Strauss and Pochi are also highly recommended. See Strauss, J. S., and Pochi, P. E.: Handbuch der Haut und Geschlechtskrankheiten. Ergänzungswerk 1/1 S. Springer, New York, 1968, pp. 184–223.

Three types of sebaceous follicle, adult beard, vellus and sebaceous, are present in skin, and only one, the sebaceous follicle, participates in the development of acne. The fully developed beard hair keeps its duct swept clean of debris and bacteria, and the vellus follicle, containing a puny hair, functions principally in contributing to the surface oiliness of the skin. As acne progresses and vellus hairs become displaced, however, they may act as foreign bodies and contribute significantly to inflammatory nodules.

Classification of Acne

In the older medical literature, there were many designations for the different phases of acne, and considerable confusion resulted. A simple designation of grades of severity has been suggested and has proved generally useful.* Grade I is comedonal acne, with less than 30 comedones, usually confined to the forehead and cheeks; Grade II acne consists of comedones and a very occasional small pustule; Grade III is characterized by comedones and inflamed pustules, with an occasional inflamed cyst and lesions on the face and upper trunk; and Grade IV (acne conglobata) consists of large pustules, cysts, connecting sinuses, inflamed nodules and a relentless course with certainty of significant scarring. (The term *conglobata* means simply "nodule" and is not entirely appropriate and inclusive. It has persisted through long usage).

With enlargement and increased secretion of the sebaceous glands at puberty comedones form. These are of two types, open and closed. The open one is the familiar blackhead with a fairly large orifice and a black melanin-tipped, worm-like expressible content of sebum, keratin, *Propionibacterium acnes* and yeasts. This lesion is of little importance other than cosmetic, although it may occasionally give rise to a ring of mild inflammation around individual lesions. Expression of the contents with a comedone extractor removes the peripheral portion of the plug and improves the cosmetic appearance. The blackhead returns in full flower within a month or so, however.

Another type of open comedone, a rather conspicuous one, is seen on the malar prominences of older persons as the result of chronic exposure to sunlight through the years. Expression of these may be desirable, although considerable pressure is often necessary. The use of an abrasive material or device (Buf-Puf, 3M Co.) may be tried. These lesions are of no significance or relation to true acne.

The primary lesion of acne is the "closed comedone." These are small cystic collections of sebum, keratinous material, and *P. acnes* in an epithelial sac. They are hardly visible to the naked eye, as is the almost micro-

---

*Pillsbury, D. M., Shelley, W., and Kligman, A. M.: Dermatology. W. B. Saunders Co., Philadelphia, 1956.

scopic opening to the surface. The closed comedone is the starting gate of inflammatory acne. The epithelial wall of the sac and canal shows variations in its structure, some of which undoubtedly relate to the wall's integrity and, possibly, to its resistance to enzymes and toxins of an as yet undetermined nature. The numerous *P. acnes* are not, apparently, destructive or toxic to the epithelial wall of the sac.

The Inflammatory Process

The sebaceous piliary apparatus becomes infused with inflammation, and rupture of the epithelial sac occurs, either in minute isolated form or more extensively, with migration of the contents into the surrounding dermis. This inevitably initiates inflammation of varying degrees. One certain fact stands out: sebum is extremely toxic to dermal structures. One of us (DMP) observed an experiment carried out by J. S. Strauss, in which an emulsion of sebum was injected into the normal skin of a male subject. The resultant inflammation was prompt, severe and alarming. There can be no question that sebum finds an extremely inhospitable reception in dermal tissue.

In the patient with acne, rupture of the comedonal sac produces a variety of inflammatory changes ranging from small pustules and inflamed papules to large fluctuant inflamed cysts, some of them interconnecting. The distribution of lesions may increase greatly, with involvement of the neck, shoulders, chest and upper back. Such lesions may drain from many openings, soiling clothing and bedclothing. As the process persists, extensive and profound structural disarrangements of the pilosebaceous apparatus occur, along with eventual scarring. At the end stage, clusters of large open comedones frequently develop. Foreign body granulomas appear frequently and persist for protracted periods.

Treatment

The therapeutic management of acne, particularly Grades III and IV, requires careful clinical judgment in the selection of topical and systemic treatment and, all important, patience on the part of both doctor and patient. Unfortunately, there is no treatment that will check acne with prompt regularity. Selection of the type of treatment will depend upon the severity of the disease and, to some extent, the patient's reaction to it. In this age of constant emphasis on the vital importance of cosmetic perfection, many youngsters, particularly females, regard even a mild comedone acne as an utter tragedy.

Topical Treatment

CHEMICAL COMPOUNDS.   The number of compounds employed in the past is remarkable, and many of them are fading from the therapeutic scene. Combinations of sulphur and resorcin predominated for decades. Others have included hexachlorophene, germicidal soaps, chlorhydroxyquinoline, sodium sulfacetamide, various wetting agents, hydrocortisone and abrasive compounds. Benzoyl peroxide in 5 to 10 per cent strength is now widely used, and 3 to 5 per cent salicylic acid in 20 per cent ethyl and 80 per cent propylene alcohol is useful. Erythromycin solution in a concentration of 2 to 5 per cent is useful in pustular acne but must be freshly prepared and kept under refrigeration.

The most striking advance in the topical treatment of acne in the past decade has been the demonstration that retinoic acid (tretinoin) solution in a strength of 0.1 to 0.01 per cent has marked comedolytic effects. It is primarily of value in acne Grades I and II but may be tried for its contributory effect in more severe pustular acne.*

WASHING.   Many patients with acne believe that the disease results from dirt and superficial infection and try to combat it with frequent washing, often in a compulsive way. They should understand that any surface lipids removed are rapidly replaced and that washing will have no effect on bacteria below the tip of the comedo.

X-RAY THERAPY.   Discussion of this mode of therapy is certain to arouse vigorous discussion, often rancorous, for and against. Thirty to 40 years ago, almost every patient with significant acne was advised to have superficial x-ray therapy, usually given in courses of 8 or 10 exposures of 50 to 75 R each. The calibration of many units was uncertain, the protection of the thyroid variable and the total amount of irradiation carried beyond the supposedly safe limit of 1000 R. The senior author observed many cases of x-ray atrophy and epithelioma in patients treated in that era, but they have now largely disappeared from the clinical scene. With the improvement of other methods of therapy, x-ray treatment for benign dermatoses has declined.

Starting in the late 1960's, it was reported that patients who had received x-ray therapy for benign diseases of the head and neck developed

---

*In 1978, a special committee of the American Academy of Dermatology issued a communication based on the finding that epithelial tumors develop in albino hairless mice exposed to various combinations of ultraviolet radiation and locally applied retinoic acid. This effect was variable. Its relevance to human experience is uncertain. In more than seven years of widespread use of retinoic acid in man, no similar sequence of events has been reported. Nevertheless, the following restrictions should be observed. (1) Patients using topical retinoic acid products should strictly adhere to the precautions contained in the drug package insert, which states: "Exposure to sunlight, including sun lamps, should be minimized during the use of this product and patients with sunburn should be advised not to use the product until fully recovered because of heightened susceptibility to sunlight as a result of the use of retinoic acid. Patients who may be required to have considerable sun exposure due to occupation should exercise particular caution. Other weather extremes, such as wind and cold, also may be irritating to patients under treatment with retinoic acid.". (2) Furthermore, patients whose skin is genetically predisposed to the development of sunlight-induced skin cancer or who exhibit unusual susceptibility to skin damage from sunlight should be particularly careful to protect themselves from sunlight exposure while using retinoic acid products.

thyroid tumors many years after such therapy was given.* The number of thyroid tumors reported to date has been relatively small, and conclusions are uncertain. The reports are disconcerting, to say the least, however, and wide distribution to the lay public has produced considerable concern.

A large-scale epidemiologic survey of this problem is needed but probably impossible in view of the decades between the treatment of acne and the detection of a thyroid tumor. The matter must, for the time being, remain very much *sub judice.*

Systemic Therapy

ANTIBACTERIAL.   The availability of antibiotics that can gain entrance to the sebaceous apparatus has afforded a significant advance in the treatment of pustular Grades III and IV acne. Tetracycline is the usual drug of choice, in an initial dose of 1 gm. daily, continued at this level for 2 to 4 weeks and then reduced gradually to 250 mg. daily if some favorable response is noted. Continuance at a low level for several months is usually necessary. Adverse effects at this level are uncommon, though occasional. Monilial overgrowth and vaginitis may be encountered. Erythromycin is an excellent alternative. Sulfonamides are relatively ineffective and occasionally productive of severe reactions. Dapsone (DDS) is an alternative drug, but it should be used with full realization of its adverse hematologic potential.

SURGICAL MEASURES.   In inflamed cystic acne lesions, there is a strong temptation to incise the lesion adequately, as with a furuncle. This ordinarily fails; the cyst promptly recurs. A better procedure is to withdraw as much of the contents as possible through a needle and then inject triamcinolone acetonide in a strength of 2.5 mg. per ml. This is often followed by a prompt flattening out of the cyst, although the procedure may have to be repeated two or three times for individual lesions.

ENDOCRINE THERAPY.   Estrogen suppresses sebaceous gland acne, although unwarranted feminizing effects will be noted in males, and such treatment is impractical. Treatment of acne with a contraceptive pill achieved considerable vogue for a time, but we would estimate that it is not widely used for acne per se at present. We have not been greatly impressed with its efficacy.

DIET.   This has been a favorite point of attack in acne. Adolescents are regularly given long lists of foods to be avoided, usually containing foods that the patients crave and often, in addition, essential nutrients. We are unconvinced that diet plays any significant role in the course of

---

*Useful references on the effects or current use of x-ray therapy in dermatologic practice are: Albright, E. C., and Allday, R. W.: Thyroid carcinoma after radiation therapy for adolescent acne vulgaris. JAMA *199*:260 (1967); DeGroot, L., and Paloyan, E.: Thyroid carcinoma and radiation. A Chicago endemic. JAMA *225*:487 (1973); and Goldschmidt, H.: Ionizing radiation therapy in dermatology; current use in the United States and Canada. *In* A Review of the Use of Ionizing Radiation for the Treatment of Benign Diseases. U.S. Department of Health, Education and Welfare Publication No. 78-8043, 1977, pp. 17–27.

acne. If a food, such as chocolate or milk is suspected, abstinence for 2 or 3 weeks, followed by deliberate ingestion may be tried, though the results may be equivocal. A striking feature of stringent diet exclusion in acne in many cases is that it is a source of mother-child conflict.

SUNLIGHT AND ULTRAVIOLET (UV) LIGHT.   In individuals who tan, acne generally improves after repeated exposure to summer sun. This is less frequently the case in redheads and blondes, in whom exacerbations may be noted. We are unimpressed with the beneficial effects of articial UV sources on acne.

13-CIS-RETINOIC ACID.   Recent studies have demonstrated that the administration of 13-cis-retinoic acid by mouth produces a reduction of the rate of secretion from the sebaceous glands. It has also produced favorable clinical effects in a limited number of patients with severe acne.

Recent evidence indicates that an oral synthetic retinoid, 13-cis-retinoic acid, is useful in the management of patients with severe acne. Fourteen patients with very severe treatment-resistant cystic acne were treated with 13-cis-retinoic acid in an average dosage of 2 mg./kg./day. Thirteen of the fourteen patients were reported to have total clearance of their disease; the fourteenth was reported to have 75 per cent improvement. Of great significance is the fact that most of these patients had prolonged remission after the completion of a 16-week course of therapy. The full potential mechanism of action of this drug is unknown at present. It is known, however, that retinoids can affect epithelial tissues, and chemical changes that occur in surface lipids of patients treated with 13-cis-retinoic acid indicate that there is a profound suppression of sebaceous gland activity. Such suppression has been confirmed in unpublished reports. 13-cis-retinoic acid definitely holds great promise as a therapeutic agent, but additional trials are necessary to determine the safety as well as the correct therapeutic dosage of the drug.*

Variants of Acne

There are several syndromes that although they simulate severe acne, represent deviations from the normal course of that disease. Brief summaries of several of these follow.

Folliculitis.   (Bockhart's impetigo) is a perifollicular staphylococcal infection that may be taken for a comedo but has no relation to acne.

---

*This brief summary of recent studies of 13-cis-retinoic acid was supplied by Dr. J. S. Strauss, Chairman and Director of the Department of Dermatology of the University of Iowa School of Medicine. References for it are listed at the end of the chapter.

Milia.   These are small superficial keratinous cysts of cosmetic significance only. They are easily removed by a small scalpel opening and expression with a comedo extractor.

Drug Eruptions.   Iodides are capable of exacerbating acne or producing an acne-like eruption. The local lesions can become severely inflammatory.

Pseudofolliculitus.   This condition, seen principally in blacks, is the result of hair tips curving back into the skin just before reaching the surface. The condition may be helped by tedious removal of the ingrown hair, but the best treatment is to nurture a beard.

Trauma-induced Acne.   A common source of worsening mild or severe acne is trauma. In young girls with long fingernails, a minimal acne may be transformed into a scarring eruption by constant picking of the skin. This may become a traumatic habit tic that is very difficult to reverse. At the other end of the acne scale, severe widespread Grade IV acne may be produced by rubbing trauma, athletic gear, heavy work clothing, back packs and so on.

Tropical Acne.   This is a widespread Grade IV acne that develops in persons suddenly transferred to a hot muggy climate. They may or may not have had significant acne previously. The only relief to be obtained is transfer to a cool, low humidity environment.

Keloids and Hypertrophic Scars.   Either of these conditions may develop after acne, though rarely on the face (see Chapter 21).

The Acne Triad.   Rarely in a patient with significant acne, a highly characteristic triad develops. It consists of Grade IV acne, a widespread deep chronic folliculitis of the scalp and hidradenitis of the axillae and anogenital region. All this may occasionally be accompanied by a pilonidal cyst.

Pyoderma Faciale.   This is an explosive type of Grade IV acne affecting young white females. Vigorous, prompt therapy is indicated if severe scarring is to be avoided. Its precise relation to true acne is uncertain.

ROSACEA

The tendency of individuals to flush in the areas of the forehead, nose and malar prominences varies greatly. In some individuals, the flush becomes permanent and rather marked, occurring sometimes as early as the twenties but more commonly at 40 or more. This may or may not be accompanied by pustule formation, which is occasionally explosive and severe. Pustules in the tense skin of the nose may be quite tender and bothersome. A late effect is marked thickening and permanent redness of the skin of the nose, with occasional development of rather prominent telangiectatic superficial venules (rhinophyma).

Treatment

The treatment of rosacea is quite similar to that used in acne. Antibiotic therapy in small doses may be successful in controlling pustules. The response of the erythema to systemic corticosteroid therapy is occasionally quite striking, but usually temporary. Such therapy is not advised. Extended topical corticosteroid therapy is *not* recommended.

In addition to the usual topical medicaments, pustular flare-ups in rosacea may respond to the application of hot Vleminckx's solution at bedtime. Response of rosacea to exposure to sunlight is variable. Diet is sometimes a significant factor in this disease. Patients may note definite flare-ups after the ingestion of coffee, alcoholic beverages, very hot or very cold drinks or highly spiced foods. This must be determined by trial. The emotional component in flushing of the face is undoubted and may be a significant factor in rosacea. The most important complication of rosacea is rosacea keratitis. Fortunately, this is rare.

MILIARIA

Miliaria can be an annoying scourge for people living in an environment that produces excessive sweating. It is due to a blockage of sweat ducts. This may follow some superficial inflammation of the skin, as in dermatitis or the application of adhesive tape or prolonged wet compresses. If the blockage occurs at the very opening of the sweat duct, all that is noted is a clear small vesicle that causes no symptoms. This is regularly seen in persons who sustain a sunburn and then exercise vigorously a day or two later. (Fig. 8–7).

When the blockage of the sweat duct occurs a little farther down, sweat escapes from the duct into the surrounding tissue and produces inflammation. This is true miliaria rubra (prickly heat). When the individual sweats, it produces very marked itching, which is relieved only if a cool environment, such as an air conditioned room, is available. A cool shower or tub bath may be helpful. No external treatment is of particular value, but a shake lotion containing 0.1 per cent menthol and 1 per cent camphor may be soothing. If there are severely inflamed areas, topical corticosteroid preparation may be tried. In occasional cases, a short course of systemic corticosteroids may be indicated.

In occasional instances, particularly after a prolonged severe drug eruption, such as is seen in patients with atabrine dermatitis, the blockage may occur much deeper down near the sweat gland itself. In persons with involvement of a high proportion of ducts, tolerance to heat and vigorous exercise may be significantly diminished.

REFERENCES

Peck, G. L., Olsen, T. G., Yoder, F. W., Strauss, J. S., Downing, D. T., Pandya, M., Butkus, D., and Arnaud-Battandier, J.: Prolonged remission of cystic and conglobate acne with 13-cis-retinoic acid. N. Engl. J. Med. 300:229–333, 1979.

Strauss, J. S., Peck, G. L., Olsen, T. G., Downing, D. T., and Windhorst, D. B.: Alteration of skin lipid composition by oral 13-cis-retinoic acid: Comparison of pretreatment and treatment values. J. Invest. Dermatol. 70:223, 1978.

Strauss, J. S., Peck, G. L., Olsen, T. G., Downing, D. T., and Windhorst, D. B.: Sebum composition during oral 13-cis-retinoic acid administration. J. Invest. Dermatol. 70:228, 1978.

Strauss, J. S.: Unpublished data.

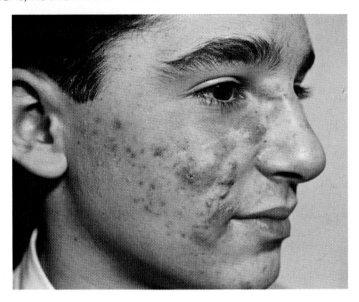

Figure 8–1. Grade III acne

Various lesions of acne are present—comedones, small superficial pustules and inflamed cysts. The response to systemic antibiotic therapy and injection of a corticosteroid into the cysts was prompt, though this is by no means always the case.

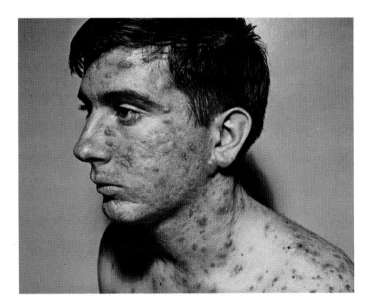

Figure 8–2. Grade IV acne

Extensive, longstanding lesions of face, neck and upper trunk. Note large cyst near lobule of ear, a common location. The response to systemic antibiotic therapy was indifferent. Acne of this chronicity and extent may have severe adverse psychologic effects.

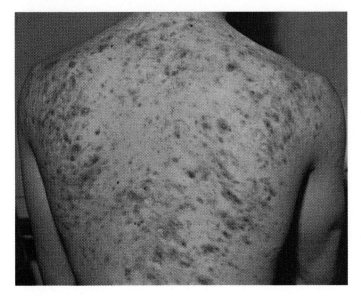

Figure 8–3. Acne

Back lesions of varying severity. With frankly pustular lesions the outlook for response to systemic antibiotic therapy, even in modest doses, is reasonably good.

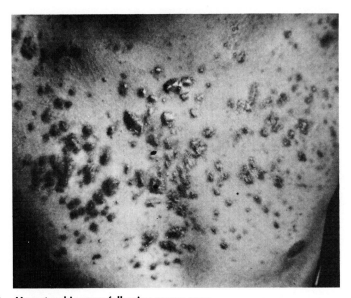

Figure 8–4. Hypertrophic scars following severe acne

Scarring is extensive in this patient following resolution of his active inflammatory lesions.

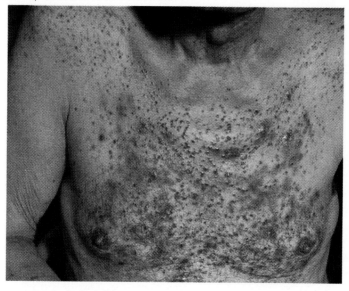

Figure 8–5. Steroid acne

Acneiform eruption following prolonged steroid therapy in patient with multiple myeloma. A relatively uncommon reaction. A clinically similar eruption may be seen in workers exposed to chlorinated hydrocarbons.

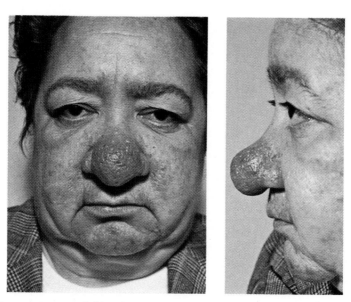

Figure 8–6. Rosacea and rhinophyma

May be improved by dermabrasion, but only by operators with some talent for sculpture.

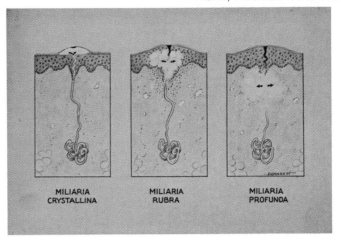

Figure 8–7.   Types of miliaria

The clinical type of miliaria is determined by the depth of the sweat duct obstruction. Miliaria crystallina is noninflammatory. The only certain method of treatment is a cool environment. The obstruction in miliaria profunda may be irreversible.

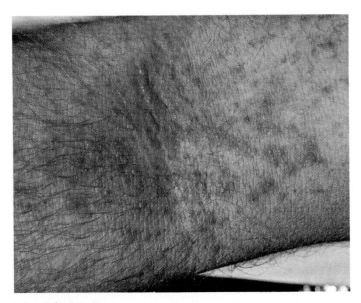

Figure 8–8.   Miliaria rubra

Exposure to a hot environment produces severe, unremitting, sleep-interfering pruritus.

9

Papulosquamous Eruptions and Connective Tissue Diseases

PAPULOSQUAMOUS ERUPTIONS

Among the skin diseases frequently encountered are a group that have little in common other than appearing in lesions that are papular and that show varying degrees of scaling, hence papulosquamous.

PSORIASIS

This disease affects from 1 to 2 per cent of the adult white population in varying degree. It may appear at any time from infancy to the seventh decade, though it is most common in early adult life. Its severity varies from one or two patches in the scalp or on the elbows, to widespread scaling plaques, to a generalized scaling erythema. Its cosmetic implications in many patients are significant, so much so that it may be classified among the "socially disabling" diseases. When it occurs on the palms or soles, the fissuring that occurs may frequently be quite disabling physically. In some instances the involvement of intertriginous areas, particularly in the anogenital region, is highly uncomfortable because of itching and fissuring.

The essential lesion of psoriasis is a papule or large plaque that is ordinarily sharply marginated from the surrounding normal skin. In its chronic form it has a distinctive silvery-white scale, which when dislodged, shows characteristic small bleeding points. In probably 75 per cent of cases, psoriasis has a distribution pattern that includes the scalp, the external ears, the elbows and knees and the trunk. In some cases the pattern of distribution is that of seborrheic dermatitis, involving particularly the scalp, the area behind the ears and the axillae and anogenital regions. Mixtures of these two distribution patterns are not uncommon.

A history of psoriasis in a blood relative will be obtained in about one-third of patients. In some instances several members of a family may

136

be affected. The exact genetic mode of transmission has not been established.

Involvement of the nails is common in psoriasis and may easily be confused with a fungal infection. In occasional instances the nail involvement is predominant, with minimal evidence of psoriasis elsewhere.

A distressing accompaniment of psoriasis is an arthritis which is similar in many respects to rheumatoid arthritis. The most commonly involved joints are the distal phalangeal. Instances are seen in which the course of the arthritis appears to correspond to exacerbation and remissions of the skin manifestations, though this is by no means invariable.

The morphology of the psoriatic lesions varies considerably, from small papules to larger plaques, sometimes with the development of striking circinate and gyrate lesions. Psoriasis affecting the palms and soles frequently escapes proper diagnosis for a long period of time. However, here again the lesions follow the general rule of being sharply circumscribed and usually most marked in areas of greatest trauma. Painful fissuring of such lesions is characteristic. Psoriasis occasionally affects the palms and soles in erythematous plaques studded with sterile pustules.

Itching is not a frequent symptom in most patients with psoriasis. However, there are exceptions in the form of plaques in the scalp, particularly in the occipital region, in which there may be a combination of psoriasis and localized neurodermatitis. Involvement of the anogenital region is frequently accompanied by itching of considerable severity. In areas that are scratched there may be extension of the lesions of psoriasis. The normal skin of such patients is susceptible to the development of a psoriatic lesion following any type of trauma.

Patients with psoriasis are usually otherwise healthy, with the exception of occasional arthritis. The factors that contribute to the onset of the disease or to exacerbations are uncertain. However, flare-ups may occur after an upper respiratory infection or subsequent to a drug reaction. Psoriasis ordinarily becomes worse during cold weather, when there is little opportunity for exposure to natural sunlight. Psychosomatic factors have been invoked in psoriasis, but their influence is uncertain. Psoriasis may sometimes exacerbate with fever in widespread pustules and erythematous plaques.

Management

As in any other disease for which no completely curative treatment exists, and in which spontaneous involution is very unlikely, the management of psoriasis involves the art and sympathy of the physician, as well as his skills.

In psoriasis that is limited in extent, e.g., a little scaling of the elbows and knees, which is not particularly bothersome, no treatment other than regular washing of the skin and the application of an emollient cream is indicated. Physicians who have had extended experience with the treatment of psoriasis generally agree that oftentimes each particular method of treatment for psoriasis seems to become less effective in time, and the maintenance of a "therapeutic reserve" is to be jealously guarded. For the initial topical treatment of psoriasis, potent corticosteroid preparations lead the field by far. Small amounts of the cream should be rubbed in twice daily. If feasible, occlusion of the area with a polyethylene film at night increases the effectiveness of the cream. The addition of 2 to 3 per cent salicylic acid to corticosteroid ointment may increase its effectiveness (Harvey Blank). For lesions of the scalp a solution of a corticosteroid in propylene glycol is more cosmetically acceptable. In widespread psoriasis, the expense of topical corticosteroid preparations becomes a significant deterrent to their regular use. Regular shampooing is advisable, and preparations containing tar may sometimes seem to be more effective than ordinary soap. In the treatment of small patches of psoriasis on nonhairy skin, particularly the hands and feet, the application of a tape impregnated with flurandrenolide is useful and convenient.

Alternate topical preparations include coal tar mixtures such as 10 to 20 per cent solution of coal tar in hydrophilic cream, or 3 to 6 per cent crude coal tar in Lassar's paste. The latter preparation is understandably messy and is not particularly feasible on an outpatient basis. The addition of natural sunlight or an adequate artificial ultraviolet B light source enhances the therapeutic effects of tars (Goeckerman regimen). As an alternative, the Ingram regimen may be employed with hospitalized patients. Anthralin 0.1 to 1 per cent in an ointment or paste applied under stockinette bandages is substituted for the topical tars used in the Goeckerman regimen and may be strikingly effective in resistant cases of psoriasis.

Psoralen (8-methoxy psoralen) taken systemically and used in combination with high-energy sources of ultraviolet light A (PUVA regimen) has produced dramatic therapeutic results in psoriasis. At this time, it is still under the strict supervision of the Federal Drug Administration. The long-term effects of PUVA therapy, particularly in the forms of skin cancer and cataracts, await final determination. (See Chapter 14 for a discussion of psoriasis phototherapy.)

Systemic corticosteroid therapy is frequently rapidly effective in psoriasis, and there is a great temptation to employ it unjustifiably. Some physicians avoid such therapy completely, but in very widespread psoriasis in which there is danger of a universal erythroderma, it may become necessary. It should be undertaken, however, with the clear realization that the rebound phenomena on discontinuance of such therapy may be quite severe.

The cancer chemotherapeutic agents methotrexate and hydroxyurea have been widely used in the treatment of psoriasis. Both are very toxic and should be administered only in very threatening situations. Methotrexate should not be given to alcoholics or patients with cirrhosis. Liver biopsy before therapy and at six-month intervals during therapy is considered obligatory. Renal and hematologic status must be carefully and frequently reviewed with both drugs. Neither drug should be used to treat patients who desire progeny. Likewise, they should not be used in pregnancy since both are mutagenic and teratogenic. Dosage schedules for the treatment of psoriasis vary widely. Methotrexate 25 mg. orally once a week is suggested for the initial dose in adults. The size of subsequent doses will depend upon clinical response and toxicity. Hydroxyurea 500 mg. twice a day for 7 to 14 days is suggested initially. As with methotrexate, adjustments to therapy are based upon clinical response and toxicity.

PITYRIASIS ROSEA

This is a rather common self-limited papulosquamous disease in which the clinical features are clear-cut and easily recognizable. However, a misdiagnosis of tinea corporis is frequently made.

Pityriasis rosea is probably due to some infectious agent. Clinically the disease is characterized by the initial appearance of a single oval area with a characteristic thin scaling border and slightly yellowish discoloration of the center. This is the primary or "herald" plaque. Within a few days to two weeks other similar lesions appear, though these are usually smaller. The sites of involvement are most commonly the trunk and upper portions of the extremities, and on the trunk the longitudinal axes of the lesions tend to follow the lines of cleavage (Christmas tree arrangement). The face is not commonly involved, though this is not an invariable rule.

Symptoms from this disease are absent or mild, but there are exceptions. Occasionally the lesions may be more inflammatory. It is not contagious. Repeated attacks are very uncommon.

In the average case, and in the absence of significant symptoms, no treatment is necessary, and the disease ordinarily runs its course in from four to eight weeks, though occasionally it lasts longer. Exposure to natural sunlight is rather consistently helpful. Should there be significant inflammation and itching, limited systemic corticosteroid therapy is almost always helpful and may be given in the form of an intramuscular injection of 40 mg. of triamcinolone acetonide.

SYPHILIS (See Chapter 19)

Early syphilis may produce lesions that are very similar to other papulosquamous eruptions, but the differentiation usually presents no difficulties.

LICHEN PLANUS

This is an uncommon papulosquamous eruption in which there is frequently concomitant involvement of the mucous membranes and skin.

In some instances only the oral mucosae show lesions. The disease first appears in the form of shiny violaceous flat-topped papules occurring principally on the flexor surfaces of the wrists and arms, the trunk, mucous membranes and genitalia. The lesions are so characteristic as to be recognizable on sight by an experienced observer. Itching may be marked. The genital lesions may be confused with syphilis.

A characteristic of lichen planus is that new lesions tend to occur along scratch marks whether from itching or accidentally. The most important aspect of the disease is oral involvement, in which the lesions may persist for years and may occasionally evolve into leukoplakia and malignancy. The nails frequently show distortion in lichen planus.

Treatment.   The treatment of lichen planus is not entirely satisfactory. Corticosteroid creams may be used, and a short trial course of systemic corticosteroid therapy may be justified. A holiday in a relaxed sunny environment may be helpful. In respect to the mouth lesions, it is particularly important that irritants be avoided, including smoking or ingestion of very hot or otherwise irritating food or drink. They may respond to intralesional injections of triamcinolone acetonide.

DERMATOPHYTOSIS (See Chapter 17)

The so-called "tineas" occur most commonly in environments that are warm and moist. Lesions in the scalp and on the face, trunk and extremities are frequently papulosquamous. Skin scrapings digested with 20 per cent potassium hydroxide (KOH) are frequently diagnostic. Fungal cultures are desirable to identify pathogens and to determine drug sensitivities.

CONNECTIVE TISSUE DISEASES

Within the past two decades, there has been an increasing awareness of a large group of diseases known as collagen or connective tissue diseases. The term "collagen" is incorrect and is disappearing. "Connective tissue disease" is also a less than completely satisfactory designation, but it is in common use.

LUPUS ERYTHEMATOSUS

Of this group of diseases, lupus erythematosus (LE) has the highest incidence, though it is uncommon in respect to most other diseases affecting the skin. It is convenient and useful to divide LE into *discoid* (DLE) and *systemic* (SLE) types, though there is much to suggest that these are at opposite ends of the same basic disease spectrum.

Discoid LE.   DLE is a distinctive scaling eruption of the skin, ordinarily distributed, in decreasing frequency, to the face, scalp, ears, chest and arms. The initial lesion is a small erythematous patch that may arise spontaneously or after mild injury or overexposure to sunlight. It enlarges slowly, with a characteristic scaling border and varying degrees of atrophy at the center. A biopsy taken from the active periphery reveals a highly characteristic microscopic picture. The lesions eventually produce marked cosmetic disfigurement. In lesions of the scalp, permanent scarring alopecia is the rule.

Though patients with discoid LE usually have no overt signs or symptoms of systemic disease, certain laboratory tests may show abnormalities of varying degree. These include leukopenia and thrombocytopenia, positive rheumatoid factor test, reactive STS, increased sedimentation rate, antinuclear factors and others. If a diagnosis of LE is suspected, *it is of the utmost importance that the patient be carefully studied to determine whether or not there is significant systemic disease.* The prognosis in discoid LE is ordinarily good. Treatment is usually effective and differs from that for SLE.

TREATMENT OF DISCOID LE.   Topical corticosteroid therapy is the initial treatment of choice. One of the more potent fluorinated steroids should be selected and applied 2 to 3 times daily. Occlusion with a polyethylene film increases effectiveness, but this should not be so prolonged, i.e., many weeks, as to risk atrophy from treatment as well as from the disease. Intralesional corticosteroid injections may become necessary, using an initial strength of not greater than 2.5 mg. per ml. of triamcinolone acetonide, to avoid undue risk of atrophy. Flurandrenolide-impregnated tape is a convenient method of treating small lesions.

The second effective method of treatment of DLE is with antimalarial drugs. Chloroquine (Aralen) is the drug of choice. It is usually administered in an initial "loading" dose of 500 mg. per day for two weeks, then reduced to 250 mg. per day. A "baseline" ophthalmologic examination is indicated before chloroquine therapy is started, with frequent re-examinations thereafter if therapy is continued. The possible eye reactions include corneal deposits and progressive retinopathy, which are rarely encountered in patients with DLE who are on a moderate dose of 250 mg. per day, with rest periods of two weeks after each month or two of treatment. Other reactions to chloroquine include bleaching and other color changes in the hair and skin and occasional dermatitis.

The administration of a combination preparation containing chloroquine, hydroxychloroquine and quinacrine (Triquin) has been advised, but there is no proof of its increased efficacy, and the possibility of reactions is probably increased.

Some patients with DLE appear to be made worse by exposure to sunlight, though there are differences of opinion on the importance of this factor. Avoidance of undue exposure or, if this is unavoidable, the use of sunscreen preparations would appear advisable in most patients.

Systemic LE.   SLE is one of the most protean of all diseases of man. It may affect any organ system; hematologic or renal involvement are the most significant. The course of the disease varies from smoldering over a period of years to one of great violence and rapidity. There are dermatologic lesions of SLE in some four-fifths of all cases. The skin lesions are a reasonably accurate reflection of the activity of the disease as a whole.

The skin lesions of SLE may sometimes resemble those of the discoid type, but they seldom produce the same degree of atrophy. The rash may be diffuse, often in areas exposed to light and is erythematous at onset but may sometimes develop a dusky, rather cyanotic, tinge. Bullae and purpura may develop, particularly during acute flare-ups. A telangiectatic erythema of the thenar and hypothenar eminences is common, and splinter hemorrhages may occur under the nails. Ulceration and even gangrene of fingers may occur.

Alopecia occurs in many patients with SLE. It is not commonly of the localized round scarring type seen in DLE but a diffuse erythema, with broken-off hairs that give a characteristic scruffy unkempt appearance.

The organic signs of SLE are so numerous and varied as to defy brief summarization. Among these the renal changes are very important, and when they develop early in the course of the disease, the prognosis must be guarded. Mucous membrane lesions may occur, with purpura and painful ulceration. The heart may be involved, with pericarditis and, occasionally, a characteristic endocarditis.

Muscle pain is common in SLE, and the initial diagnosis may be arthritis. Central nervous system involvement may be signaled by epileptiform seizures or psychiatric abnormalities.

The abnormal laboratory findings in SLE are numerous, but they are sometimes equivocal in establishing a solid diagnosis. The most useful single test is the LE cell phenomenon. In the "LE prep," a characteristic cell is seen on incubation of the patient's serum or blood with leucocytes from his own buffy coat, or that of another human or of a dog. It is not, however, absolutely pathognomic of SLE. Common hematologic findings include anemia, leukopenia, thrombocytopenia, hypergammaglobulinemia, an increased erythrocyte sedimentation rate and typical immunofluorescent tissue findings. Other hematologic tests are available. Biologic false positive tests for syphilis are not uncommon.

TREATMENT OF SLE.   If ever a disease placed demands upon the full gamut of internal medicine and its subspecialties, it is SLE. The advice of physicians with broad experience with the disease should be sought. A cardinal principle is that the patient with SLE is in a brittle state medically, and that the disease may be markedly exacerbated by exposure to sunlight, by a reaction to any one of a rather lengthy list of drugs, by unusual physical stress or by interference with a focus of infection. Overmedication should be avoided. Corticosteroids, sometimes in massive doses, are the bulwark in controlling acute exacerbations of the disease.

Antimalarials and cancer chemotherapeutic agents are sometimes useful.

Other diseases classified under the connective tissue category are uncommon, though some are of great seriousness. The following is a brief summarization.

MORPHEA (LOCALIZED SCLERODERMA)

This is a distinctive disease in which one or more plaques of hardened atrophic skin develop, usually for no apparent reason, although they occasionally appear after injury. In the early stages, a plaque may have a distinctive violaceous border. The lesions may be linear and may occur on one side of the face, with atrophy of underlying muscle and bone. Intralesional corticosteroid injections may be helpful if given early in the course of the lesion.

SYSTEMIC SCLEROSIS

This was formerly termed scleroderma, but the widespread involvement of tissues other than the skin makes the term sclerosis preferable. In a high proportion of cases the onset of the disease is heralded by Raynaud's phenomenon, with increasing blanching of fingers on exposure to cold. After a period of months to years, firm hardening of the skin occurs, most commonly of the fingers, forearms, face, feet and upper trunk. This advances at a variable rate, with increasing restriction of movement, occasional calcinosis and a tendency to small ulcers, particularly of the fingers.

Systemic involvement occurs eventually, particularly of the esophagus and the rest of the G.I. tract, the lungs, heart and kidneys. Treatment, other than palliative, is unavailing.

Other connective tissue diseases are dermatomyositis and mixed or undifferentiated connective tissue disease. "Mixed" disease typically combines the major features of scleroderma and dermatomyositis. Less frequently, the features of lupus erythematosus and scleroderma occur together.

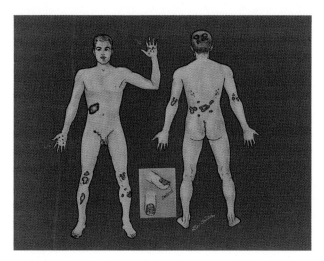

Figure 9–1.   Distribution pattern of psoriasis

These are the sites most frequently involved. Sometimes, however, the lesions are largely intriginous.

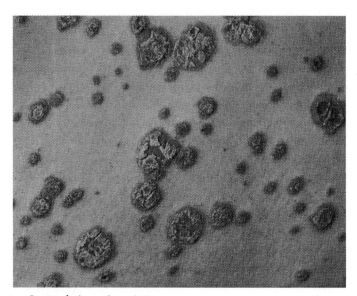

Figure 9–2.   Guttate lesions of psoriasis

In this patient many new small round lesions are developing, a rather characteristic form of flare-up of the disease. Coalescence of lesions is common, sometimes into large plaques.

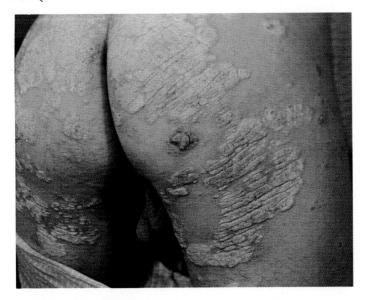

Figure 9–3.   Psoriasis and melanoma

Characteristic silvery plaques of chronic psoriasis. The tumor in the center proved to be a malignant melanoma, a pure coincidence. In the obscuring debris of a chronic dermatosis, however, early skin tumors may escape notice.

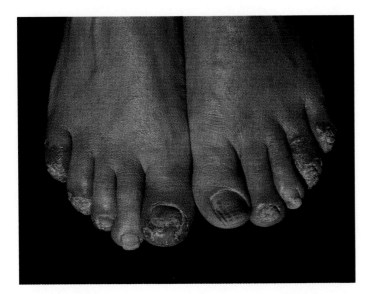

Figure 9–4.   Psoriasis of toes

Acute flare-up of psoriasis involving the toes. In the absence of evidence of the disease elsewhere, the differentiation from bacterial or *Candida* infection may be difficult; indeed, they may be secondary invaders.

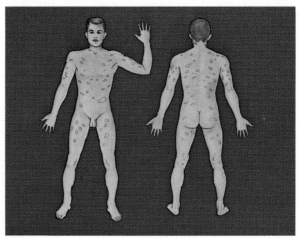

Figure 9–5.   Distribution pattern of pityriasis rosea

This distribution of lesions is seen in most cases of pityriasis rosea. Sometimes, however, the disease involves the extremities chiefly, with relatively little involvement of the trunk.

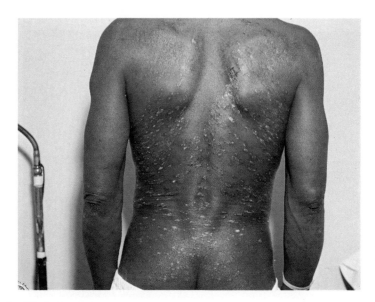

Figure 9–6.   Pityriasis rosea

This extensive papulosquamous eruption was clinically asymptomatic. The proximal distribution of the eruption along with the finding of a "herald" plaque on the chest, normal lymph nodes and normal laboratory data confirmed the diagnosis. The differential diagnosis included secondary syphilis, guttate parapsoriasis, guttate psoriasis and a drug eruption.

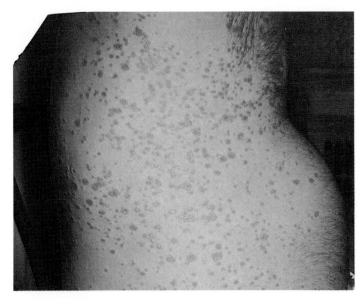

Figure 9–7.   Lichen planus

Typical papular lesions. The characteristic purplish sheen is well shown in the cross-lighted papules. Itching in lichen planus may be very marked at times.

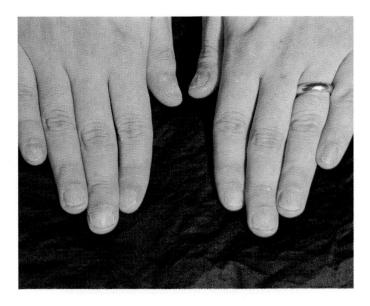

Figure 9–8.   Lichen planus of nails

The nail changes sometimes seen in patients with lichen planus are quite different from those commonly observed in psoriasis. There is little or no subungual debris, and the characteristic pitting of psoriasis is absent.

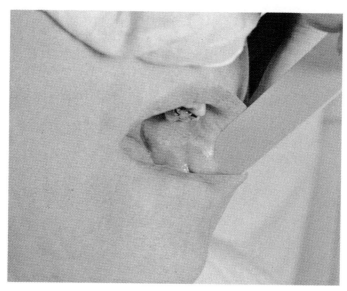

Figure 9–9. Lichen planus of buccal surface

Typical lacy-white lesions of lichen planus of the mouth. The lesions may be more extensive, and the lips may be involved. In longstanding lichen planus of the mouth, the lesions become more thickened and leukoplakic, a prerunner of possible cancer.

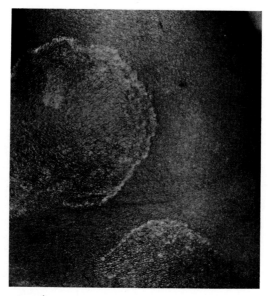

Figure 9–10. Tinea corporis

Moist, hot environments predispose to the development of extensive lesions, as may diabetes mellitus, obesity and immune deficiency. Systemic griseofulvin is considered the treatment of choice in *extensive* infections. Topical treatment with clotrimazole 1 per cent and similar compounds is reserved for more localized disease. (Courtesy of G. W. Hambrick, Jr.)

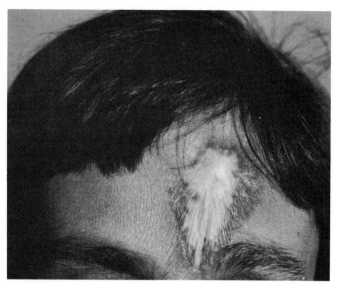

Figure 9–11.   Morphea

The "mark of the saber" designates this linear variant when it occurs on the face. If it occurs in the growing child, dystrophy of the underlying bones may occur. Rarely it may involve one side of the face to produce hemiatrophy.

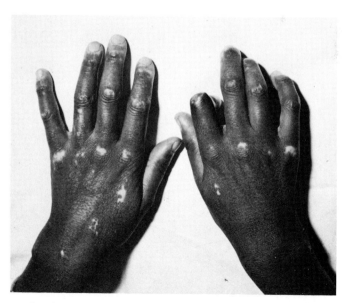

Figure 9–12.   Scleroderma—acrosclerosis

This patient has systemic sclerosis. Her hands demonstrate the hypopigmentation and attempts at repigmentation that are frequently seen over joints where ulcerations have previously occurred. Spindling of the digits and ulceration of the finger tips are common.

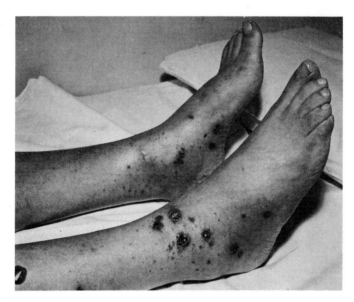

Figure 9–13.   Lupus erythematosus vasculitis

This recurrent necrotizing angiitis served as an accurate barometer of the activity of this patient's systemic disease.

10

Dermatitis and Eczema

Dermatitis of various types constitutes the largest segment of clinical dermatology.* Its course varies from brief episodes of inflammation to lifelong persistence. The clinical changes in a dermatitis tend to follow similar patterns, though with occasional marked variations.

The successive gross and microscopic changes in dermatitis, although highly variable, are as follows:

GROSS	MICROSCOPIC
1. Erythema—variable excoriation, swelling	1. Epidermal edema, separation of cells
2. Vesicles and/or bullae	2. Vesicles
3. Oozing	3. Rupture of vesicles and bullae
4. Thickening and crusting, lichenification, scaling	4. Thickening of cellular and horny layers
	5. Acanthosis and hyperkeratosis

The various types of dermatitis may be difficult to distinguish from each other microscopically, although chronic forms often have a heavy dermal cellular infiltrate. A reasonably accurate classification of various types of dermatitis is helpful in their management. The principal subdivisions follow.

CONTACT DERMATITIS

Reactions to external agents may be due to their primary irritant capacity, e.g., a material that will produce inflammation in anyone's skin if applied in sufficient concentration, or to an allergic sensitivity that has been acquired through repeated contacts with the material over a period of weeks or years. In the latter group, extremely low concentrations of the agent may be all that is necessary to produce a severe reaction. In general, reactions to primary irritants tend to appear within 24

---

*The most definitive and inclusive summary in English of the reaction of human skin to an extraordinary variety of externally encountered compounds will be found in Fisher, A. A.: *Contact Dermatitis.* Lea & Febiger, Philadelphia, 1973.

hours; allergic reactions may require 48 hours or several days to appear after exposure.

Compounds that have primary irritant effects on the skin include acids and alkalies in sufficient concentration, agents capable of producing defatting of the skin, e.g., kerosene and turpentine, and many industrial agents. Naturally occurring agents that produce sensitization reactions comprise a very wide variety of materials, including plants such as poison ivy and other members of this botanical group, primrose, chrysanthemum and many others. Sap from certain trees may produce sensitization, e.g., the Japanese lacquer tree, mahogany, white pine and others. Citrus fruits, onions and celery are some of the sensitizing fruits and vegetables handled by cooks and housewives.

There are numerous industrial agents, including paraphenylenediamine, chromate and nickel salts and others, that can cause sensitization. Many topical therapeutic agents can produce allergic sensitivity. The most common of these include penicillin, neomycin, some antihistamines and phenothiazines. Cosmetics, such as hair dyes and sprays, various hair tonics, deodorants and antiperspirants and depilatories, are a common source of allergic sensitivity reaction. Some individuals may react to material in their clothing, including wool particularly and synthetic fibers, leather and its components, dyes and elastic and supportive material in undergarments. Household contactants constitute another source of reactions, including those from detergents, polishes, waxes, metals and other agents.

Patch testing with a "scout" or "standard test" tray is a useful procedure when thorough questioning and observation of the patient yields no clue to a likely allergen in a possible contact dermatitis. In one large study, 4000 patients with eczema of various types were tested in 5 European clinics. Of 281 women with contact dermatitis, half had a positive patch test. The responsible allergens in order of frequency were balsams, nickel, various medicaments, cobalt, rubber, chromate, benzocaine and paraphenylenediamine.* It is extremely important that compounds of unknown primary irritant or allergenic capacity be applied with caution.

Many lists of substances for patch test trays are available. A representative list follows.**

1. Nickel sulfate 2.5 per cent aqueous
2. Ethylenediamine 1 per cent
3. Paraphenylenediamine 1 per cent
4. Benzocaine 5 per cent

---

*Calnan, C. D., Bandman, H. J., Cronin, E., et al.: Hand dermatitis in housewives. Br. J. Dermatol. *82*:543, (1970).

**From Fisher, A. A.: Contact Dermatitis. Lea & Febiger, Philadelphia, 1973, p. 46. (Modified from North American Contact Dermatitis Group)

5. Paraben mixture 15 per cent (5 per cent each of methyl, ethyl and propyl)
6. Thimerosal (Merthiolate) 0.1 per cent
7. Ammoniated mercury 1 per cent
8. Lanolin (as is)
9. Formaldehyde 2 per cent aqueous
10. Mercaptobenzothiazole 2 per cent
11. Tetramethylthiuram disulfide 2 per cent
12. Potassium dichromate .025 per cent aqueous
13. Turpentine 10 per cent in olive oil
14. Neomycin sulfate 20 per cent

When feasible, the compound is best mixed into petrolatum. The compound may be conveniently applied under an ordinary plastic bandage and kept in place for a "reading" at 48 hours unless a sharp reaction has intervened. In patients with adhesive tape sensitivity, Dermicel or Blenderm brand tape may be used, although both contain acrylic adhesives. The patient should be instructed to remove any patch that is producing a significant reaction. In patients receiving systemic corticosteroid therapy, reactions to patch tests are little affected. Topical steroid therapy at the site may completely obliterate the reaction, however.

Clinical Symptoms and Signs

Contact dermatitis is most frequently seen on exposed portions of the skin, e.g., face, neck, hands and forearms. In individuals wearing more abbreviated dress, the sites of involvement may be much more extensive. Reactions to various items of clothing, e.g., footgear and undergarments, may involve covered areas. In poison ivy dermatitis the antigen is frequently transferred by the hands to other areas, particularly the genitalia.

The severity of contact dermatitis varies greatly, from simple erythema and scaling, which may disappear without treatment in a few days, to a severe bullous erythematous eruption, which may progress to superficial erosions and may be vulnerable to bacterial infection and untoward reactions to applied medication. *Itching is a constant feature in allergic contact dermatitis.*

Treatment

As previously mentioned, recognition of the offending agent is essential in the management of contact dermatitis. No amount of treatment will prevent further reactions if exposure to the offending substance is continued. Frequently, a mild contact dermatitis can be rapidly cured if a potent corticosteroid cream is applied. This should be at least the equivalent of 1 per cent hydrocortisone. Wet, cool compresses or soaks with physiologic saline or Burow's solution are often soothing. The symptoms may be relieved to some extent by puncturing the bullae with curved scissors or scalpel and allowing the serous exudate to drain. Under no circumstances should the protective roof of the blister be cut away. Occlusive dressings should be avoided. Systemic corticosteroid therapy is a mainstay in severe acute contact dermatitis and, in short courses, offers very little physiologic risk. Prednisone or its equivalent is recommended in an initial daily dose of 40 to 60 mg. It should be continued for 3 or 4 days and then reduced to zero within 2 to 3 weeks. Careful observation for evidence of secondary bacterial infection is necessary, followed by administration of an appropriate systemic antibiotic if indicated. The topical application of antibiotics is not recommended in the management of contact dermatitis.

Calamine and similar lotions have rather lost their vogue in the treatment of acute contact dermatitis, but they may be used if nothing else is available. As the eruption becomes dry and less acute, hydrophilic cream USP or an equivalent bland preparation may be adequate. Boric acid soaks and compresses are not recommended because of neurotoxicity from absorption or accidental ingestion.

In a recurrent acute or chronic dermatitis suspected of being caused by a contactant, a very searching study may be necessary to pinpoint the offending substance. The history in respect to possible exposures must be particularly detailed, and the patient questioned and requestioned. In a dermatitis suspected of being related to the patient's occupation, the patient may have to stay away from his work for a period of up to 2 weeks. In chronic dermatitis, an improvement within this period may not be immediately apparent. Conducting patch tests may become advisable, using either "scout trays" of commonly encountered sensitizers or materials to which the patient is known to be exposed. Such testing should, however, be carried out after subsidence of the acute dermatitis, and *by a physician experienced in the procedure*. Severe reactions may result if too high concentrations of the irritants or sensitizers are used. The objective is to reproduce the patient's disease in miniature only.

Attempts to hyposensitize persons who have allergic contact sensitivity by oral administration or by injecting the responsible allergen usually result in failure. If this is attempted, the allergen must be administered over a period of months and in as large a total dose as can be tolerated to achieve even a moderate degree of success. In some patients who sustain repeated attacks of contact dermatitis, a degree of hyposensitization, called hardening, may occur.

ATOPIC DERMATITIS

This type of eczema is the most chronic and recurrent of the dermatitic group. Its course is highly unpredictable. Individuals with significant atopic dermatitis are rarely fit for military duty and react badly to various environmental or stressful situations.

Atopic dermatitis is usually first noted in the neonatal period. It may disappear at age 2 or thereabouts. During childhood it may be accompanied or replaced by various other manifestations of atopy, e.g., hay fever, rhinitis, asthma and rarely urticaria. After infancy the eczema usually assumes a characteristic distribution to the face, neck and antecubital and popliteal regions.

Itching is an outstanding characteristic of atopic eczema; in fact, the changes seen — thickening, color changes and scaling — are largely the result of almost unremitting rubbing and scratching. Fissures commonly develop, especially about the ears, neck and hands, and these are subject to low grade or acute infection. Atopic dermatitis fortunately disappears in the late teens or twenties in many individuals, though no absolute prediction in this regard can be made.

The single most important complication of atopic dermatitis is a generalized infection from the virus of herpes simplex or cowpox vaccine. This may result in a very severe febrile illness, with an extensive eruption resembling severe chickenpox or smallpox. The complication may be lethal. For this reason, persons with *active atopic dermatitis should not be vaccinated against smallpox*, nor should they be exposed to individuals with a cold sore (herpes simplex).

Atopic dermatitis is subject to exacerbation from a variety of factors, including prolonged nervous tension, contact of the skin with scratchy materials (particularly wool, continuing exposure to cold, inadequate hygiene and inability to apply regularly such topical medicaments as may be indicated. Many atopic patients have a dry (ichthyotic) skin that has a low tolerance to cold and low humidity. Atopic dermatitis usually improves in a summer environment and with exposure to sunlight. A summer stay at the seashore is often very helpful. However, a hot muggy environment induces increased sweating and secondary miliaria (prickly heat), which may increase itching acutely.

Treatment

The management of atopic dermatitis cannot be summarized in a few sentences. It consists of a selected potpourri of various topical and systemic medicaments, attempts to mitigate contributory factors, particularly those in the environment, and supportive psychotherapy. Formal psychotherapy, in the absence of specific indications, is disappointing.

The principal helpful measures are:

Topical Corticosteroid Therapy. This includes any approved cream or ointment with an anti-inflammatory equivalency of 1 per cent hydrocortisone or more. These must be applied regularly, at least 2 or 3 times daily. Their effectiveness is sometimes increased by covering the area of application at night with polyethylene film (Saran Wrap), but this sometimes induces increased sweating and may not be well tolerated.

Systemic Antihistaminics and Antipruritics. Any approved antihistaminic compound may be tried. Occasional good responses are noted, but these are highly irregular. The same may be said for the various antipruritics available.

Simple Bland Greasy Preparations. These are often nearly as effective as expensive corticosteroid creams. These include ordinary petrolatum, hydrophilic ointment USP, zinc oxide or Lassar's paste. Solution of coal tar 10 per cent, or 0.1 per cent menthol and 1 per cent camphor may be added. A 1 to 3 per cent concentration of ichthammol in zinc oxide paste is an old and sometimes useful remedy. Castellani's paint, applied once daily, is sometimes effective on fissures.

Systemic Corticosteroid Therapy. This is extremely effective, though *almost always temporarily*, in atopic dermatitis. It should be reserved for extensive and disabling involvement and only after careful consideration. Treatment may sometimes best be given in the form of intramuscular triamcinolone acetonide, or its equivalent, in an adult dose of 40 mg. every 3 to 4 weeks. An annoying side effect of such therapy in females is metrorrhagia and menorrhagia in approximately 10 per cent of cases. During such therapy, continuing efforts to control recurrences by other means should be made. The undesirable physiologic consequences of corticosteroid therapy when extended beyond a few weeks must always be kept in mind. Suspension of such treatment should always be gradual because the consequence of sudden withdrawal may be a severe exacerbation of the disease.

Scratch and Intradermal Tests. Performed on patients with atopic dermatitis, such tests frequently yield a high percentage of positive reactions, particularly to impure and uncertain allergens, such as extracts of house dust. Such positive reactions rarely have any etiologic significance insofar as the dermatitis is concerned, and attempts at hyposensitization by a long series of injections are quite useless and indeed carry some element of risk. Such therapy is still widely employed.

STASIS DERMATITIS

Stasis dermatitis is a common and often chronic penalty of venous insufficiency, seen principally in middle age and most commonly in multiparous women. It is not commonly encountered in young individuals; however, it may be seen in individuals who have a history of thrombophlebitis of the legs.

The initial signs, which appear most frequently over the internal malleoli of the ankles, are redness and scaling, usually asymptomatic. This is a significant warning signal of more serious and disabling disease to come. The only treatment usually necessary at this stage, however, is a supportive stocking or a fairly snug anklet worn during the day. It is helpful for the patient to acquire the habit of raising the feet on a footstool or chair when sitting. Custom-fitted Jobst brand stockings are sometimes necessary to afford adequate support.

Since stasis dermatitis is essentially a problem of venous incompetence, careful evaluation is necessary. Consultation is usually advisable. Occasionally venous surgery is required in advanced or serious cases.

From the dermatologic standpoint, it is important to keep in mind that areas of stasis dermatitis are very susceptible to the development of contact sensitivity. Furacin and neomycin compounds, among others, should be avoided. If a reaction to applied medicaments occurs, it is not unusual for a generalized nummular dermatitis to develop. Local antihistaminic and anesthetic compounds should not be used. For topical treatment, dependence should be placed on relatively bland inactive creams and pastes. Ointments containing crude coal tar (2 to 5 per cent) or a tar gel are often useful.

DERMATITIS OF HANDS AND FEET (SEE CHAPTERS 5 AND 7 FOR ILLUSTRATIONS)

Inflammatory eruptions involving the hands and feet are frequently encountered in all age groups. The etiologic factors are often diverse and may be difficult to determine precisely. They include:

Fungal Infections of the Feet.   In some cases infection of the hands will occasionally appear in association. Fungal infections of the feet (most commonly of the inflammatory type) due to *Trichophyton mentagrophytes* tend to originate in the intertriginous spaces and involve the rest of the feet in vesicular patches, sometimes in very acute fashion. Such patients may have a secondary eruption of the hands, and increased sensitivity to the extract of *Trichophyton* fungi, trichophytin, may be demonstrable. One of the most common errors of dermatologic diagnosis is the assumption that any chronic or acute inflammation of the feet is due primarily to fungal infection. The index of error in this assumption is probably at least 50 per cent. In *Trichophyton rubrum* infections, the involved areas are characteristically dry and scaling, often occurring in a moccasin-type distribution on the soles and sides of the feet.

Contact Dermatitis.   In contact dermatitis of the feet, inflammation is ordinarily most marked on the surfaces of the foot in closest contact with the foot gear. The toe webs are not involved initially. A secondary dermatitis of the hands, apparently a reaction to absorbed allergens, is not uncommon. Individuals with hyperhidrosis of the feet and hands are most susceptible. The hands are by far the most common site of contact dermatitis. It may be the primary cause or become operative secondary to some prior condition. It must *always* be considered in any dermatitis of the hands.

Psoriasis. This dermatosis may involve the hands and feet, without affecting other areas of the skin. The condition is frequently not diagnosed promptly, but it may be recognized by the sharp margination of the lesions, in the form of dry plaques that tend to fissure on slight trauma. Psoriasis may occur in the form of small sterile pustules that may be extremely recurrent and resistant to treatment. Ordinarily the nails show pitting and other changes.

Acute dermatitis involving the hands or feet may be treated, as a rule, by applying corticosteroid preparations, provided a fungal infection has been ruled out. In occasional instances, in which the clinical findings are highly suggestive, a trial of oral griseofulvin therapy in a dose of at least 1 gm. daily may be justifiable. In persistent cases, however, careful mycologic and bacteriologic study is indicated, with therapy dependent upon the findings.

Soaks in saline or Burow's solution are often soothing and will remove the epithelial debris. To control episodes of marked itching, brief exposure to hot water is often temporarily helpful.

SEBORRHEIC DERMATITIS

Many individuals have a moderate degree of seborrheic dermatitis in the form of mild to severe dandruff, which can ordinarily be controlled by more frequent shampooing, either with ordinary soap or with one of the many proprietary preparations available commercially. Nothing is curative, however, though the amount of scaling may wax and wane and is commonly worse during winter months or while occlusive head gear is worn. In many cases of seborrheic dermatitis, the skin has a greasy appearance. The application of small amounts of a corticosteroid cream as a pomade after shampooing is often helpful in delaying recurrence of the dermatitis.

More extensive seborrheic dermatitis is characterized by scaling and various degrees of redness, usually in a characteristic distribution to the scalp, eyebrows and nasal folds, behind the ears, in the presternal and interscapular areas and in the folds of the axillae and anogenital region. The cause is unknown; association with psoriasis is common. In obese individuals, particularly those with diabetes, the intertriginous involvement may extend to all body folds. Such areas are very susceptible to secondary infection by bacteria and by *Candida*. Fissuring is common.

Treatment

Topical corticosteroid therapy is the most effective single method of treatment. In treating the scalp, a liquid preparation in propylene glycol is more acceptable than a cream or ointment. Preparations having an antiinflammatory effect equivalent to 0.5 to 1.0 per cent hydrocortisone are necessary.

Creams containing sulfur and salicylic acid have long been standard in the treatment of seborrheic dermatitis. The sulfur concentration is ordinarily from 3 to 5 per cent and the salicylic acid 2 or 3 per cent. Cosmetically acceptable proprietary preparations are available. These may be used as shampoos or as creams applied the night before shampooing. Selenium sulfide suspension shampoo is helpful, used once or twice weekly. Constant observation for evidence of secondary infection, particularly bacterial, must be maintained in extensive cases. If bacterial infection is suspected, even if low grade, a systemic antibiotic is ordinarily advisable. Fissures are often helped by occasional painting with Castellani's paint.

In intertriginous involvement, the role of secondary irritative factors is important, particularly in obese persons. Intertriginous folds should be thoroughly bathed, rinsed to remove all traces of soap and then scrupulously dried. The use of antibacterial soaps does not appear to offer any particular advantage. In seborrheic dermatitis occurring behind and above the ears, mechanical irritation by or sensitization to material in spectacle frames should be considered. Either plastic or metallic frames may be responsible. Otitis externa is a common companion.

Ordinarily systemic corticosteroid therapy is rapidly effective in extensive seborrheic dermatitis. The possibility of latent or overt diabetes, however, must always be considered, particularly in obese individuals of middle age or more. It is usually possible to restrict the steroid therapy to 2 or 3 weeks, or a single intramuscular injection of 40 mg. of triamcinolone may suffice. Thereafter, well-selected topical therapy is often sufficient to keep the dermatitis under control.

LOCALIZED SCRATCH DERMATITIS (LICHEN SIMPLEX CHRONICUS)

This is a very common type of eruption that is perpetuated by repeated scratching. The itching sensation stops when pain induced by the scratching occurs, but the itching recurs after varying intervals — the scratch-itch-scratch cycle. It is one of the few dermatologic diseases in which tension factors are often clearly apparent. The area of eruption is ordinarily quite well circumscribed and is characterized by thickening of the skin with a diamond-shaped lichenification and varying degrees of erythema and scaling. The sites of involvement include any area that is easily accessible, but the most common are the occipital area (particularly in women), various other portions of the scalp, the neck, hands, perianal and vulvar areas, scrotum and legs. Anal, vulvar and scrotal pruritus may be severe and unremitting, at times all-engrossing to the patient.

Lichen simplex chronicus may be anteceded or accompanied by contact dermatitis, psoriasis or seborrheic dermatitis.

Treatment

The affected patient will ordinarily readily agree that he keeps the dermatitis active by trauma. He may be assured that if scratching is prevented for 2 to 4 weeks, the inflammation will disappear. Occasionally this may be accomplished by simply occluding the lesion with surgical tape or by some other measure.

Topical corticosteroid creams are the most useful therapeutic measure. The higher concentrations of potent preparations are best. Occlusion of the area at night or even for several days continuously with polyethylene film (Saran Wrap) or a similar product often increases the effectiveness of the cream and also prevents further scratching. If this induces excessive sweating, however, the eventual result may be poor. In small circumscribed areas the intralesional injection of an insoluble corticosteroid may be followed by prolonged or permanent relief of itching. The concentration of the steroid should not be greater than 2 to 5 mg. per ml. of triamcinolone to avoid the possibility of atrophy.

Localized neurodermatitis of the anal or vulvar regions may present special etiologic factors. In the anal region external hemorrhoids or small fissures may initiate marked itching. Scrupulous anal hygiene is essential. In chronic cases the possibility of pinworms should be considered. Anal pruritus may sometimes persist for years and be very distressing.

Chronic vulvar pruritus may often be very marked. Adequate gynecologic examination should be done to rule out contributory factors such as discharge or associated vaginal moniliasis or trichomonad infection.

Systemic corticosteroid therapy will almost never be necessary in localized neurodermatitis. Occasionally, preparations containing tars, e.g., 10 per cent solution of coal tar or 0.1 per cent menthol and 1 per cent camphor in hydrophilic ointment USP, are helpful. The itching may be temporarily relieved by very hot or very cold water. Application of preparations containing benzocaine should be avoided because of the high sensitizing capacity of this compound.

NUMMULAR DERMATITIS

This is a characteristic type of eczema, composed of coin-sized patches that are distributed principally to the extensor surfaces of the extremities and to the trunk. The face is rarely involved. Chronic or acute secondary infection is common.

Nummular dermatitis tends to occur in males of middle age or older. The cause is often uncertain. There is, however, commonly a history of previous contact dermatitis or insect bites, often with scratch dermatitis and secondary infection. The individual may have had atopic dermatitis in his youth. It is a not uncommon complication of stasis dermatitis, particularly if there has been a sensitization reaction to local medication on the legs.

This type of eczema tends to be chronic and recurrent. Itching is often marked. Local treatment of whatever type is frequently not effective, and in extensive cases systemic corticosteroid therapy may be indicated.

Bacterial culture of the lesions is advisable, and if a significant pathogenic organism, particularly coagulase-positive *Staphylococcus aureus*, is isolated, systemic antibiotic therapy is frequently helpful. Topical corticosteroid therapy may be of some value, usually in the form of a lotion or liquid preparation rather than as an ointment or cream. The local application of Castellani's paint or a tar paint may help to dry up the lesions. Exposure to natural sunlight or ultraviolet therapy is useful. Systemic corticosteroid therapy may be advisable, but the lowest effective dose should be promptly established, because such therapy may have to be rather prolonged for adequate control. Various antihistaminics and mild tranquilizers may be tried. Nummular dermatitis is often distressingly recurrent, sometimes in an extensive, explosive fashion.

TOPICAL CORTICOSTEROID THERAPY

Corticosteroids have afforded the greatest advance in topical dermatologic therapy ever achieved. In properly selected inflammatory dermatoses, they often exert astonishingly rapid symptomatic and objective improvement. If the underlying etiologic factor of the dermatosis being treated can be determined and corrected, this improvement may be permanent, but if not, recurrences will be encountered.

Since the initial introduction of hydrocortisone creams and ointments into the dermatologic formulary, a parade of new, more potent compounds have become available, particularly fluorinated analogues, which proved to be unsuitable for systemic administration because of adverse mineral corticoid effects. The risks of topical corticosteroid therapy are remarkably few, however. In general, they are encountered only in certain viral infections of the skin and in any case in which the application of the steroid is prolonged and extensive.

Therapeutic Considerations

Considerations of cost of treatment become important in extensive dermatoses, particularly chronic ones. Initial trial of a low-potency, relatively inexpensive preparation, e.g., 0.5 per cent hydrocortisone, may be worthwhile. In such a trial, the patient should be told that a more potent compound, or systemic therapy, may become advisable. Costs vary widely. They are lowest for 0.5 per cent hydrocortisone ointment and highest for highly potent 0.2 per cent fluocinolone cream.

In general, ointments are more acceptable for dry, scaling dermatoses and gel vehicles for hairy areas. Creams have general cosmetic acceptance. Corticosteroid sprays are available, but in very exudative eruptions we have found them relatively ineffective, possibly because the medication is soon washed off by the serous exudate. In conditions in which the skin surface is intact, as in urticaria, topically applied corticosteroids are ineffective.

In acute extensive reactions of the skin, as in allergic contact dermatitis, there is no justification for combining systemically administered and topically applied steroids. If indicated, systemic therapy may be given initially for a short term, e.g., 1 to 2 weeks, followed by topical treatment for the "tag ends" of the rash, or possibly just by a nonmedicated bland cream.

Significant allergic or primary irritant reactions to topically applied corticosteroids are uncommon, certainly less common than in the case of many "skin remedies" available over-the-counter. In many countries, e.g., South America, topically applied steroid preparations are sold without prescription. Adverse effects usually may be traced to some ingredient of the vehicle or to application of the preparation under polyester film occlusion. The chief adverse reactions are as follows:

1. Striae and more extensive atrophy may occur, but only after weeks or months — particularly after application of the more potent fluorinated compounds and especially if occlusion is used.

2. Possible extension of the viral infections herpes virus hominis (HVH) and varicella may occur, though we have never observed an instance of this complication. It is generally agreed that steroid preparations should not be applied to HVH infections near or involving the eye.

3. Prolonged application of potent steroids to the face may bring about a circumoral rosacea-like disease, an iatrogenic rash observed only in recent years. It is slowly reversible on cessation of the steroid medication.

4. Although the authors have never observed an overt cushingoid effect from topical corticosteroid therapy, there can be no doubt that systemic absorption in significant degree may occur with widespread application over extensive areas. Special caution should be observed in the neonatal period.

5. Though we are unaware of any significant, clinically adverse vascular effects from the superficial constriction induced by steroids, we have been unwilling to employ topical steroid preparations on inflammation or ulcers in areas in which the arterial circulation is compromised. There seems no contraindication in inflammation resulting from venostasis.

6. Purpura may be encountered after prolonged application of a potent corticosteroid.

REFERENCES

Kligman, A. M., and Leyden, J. J.: Adverse effects of fluorinated steroids applied to the face. J.A.M.A. 229:60–62, 1974.

Nair, B. K. H., and Nair, C. H. K.: Clinical evaluation of desoximetasone in treatment of dermatoses and psoriasis. Int. J. of Dermatol. 14(4):277–9, 1975.

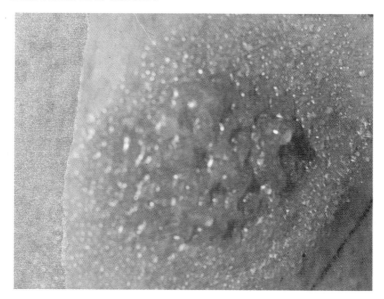

Figure 10–1. Vesicular reaction to nickel

Prolonged exposure to the antigen is required before sensitization occurs. In allergic patients, a contact patch test is frequently reactive within 48 hours, although the reaction may be delayed by 72 to 96 hours. Treatment requires the removal of costume jewelery and the use of topical steroids. Rarely, nickel-containing dental and orthopedic devices must also be removed.

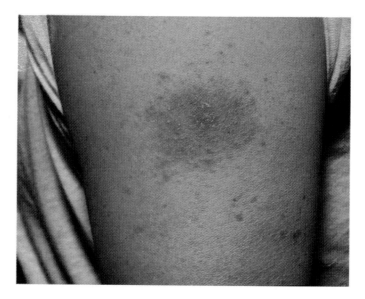

Figure 10–2. Positive patch test to extract of ragweed

Extracts of a wide variety of allergenic weeds and plants are available commercially, and testing with them is often rewarding when the history of contact is not clear-cut. Patch tests are usually reactive within 48 hours, although the response may not be appreciated up to 96 hours after antigen application.

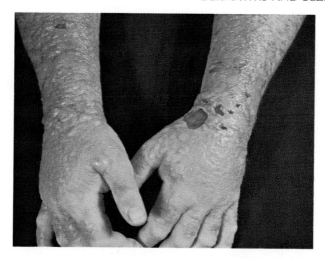

Figure 10-3.   Contact dermatitis from phenothiazine compound

This is an example of severe occupational allergic dermatitis. With many industrial chemical allergens, closed manufacturing systems are essential. The possibility of reaction may be reduced but not prevented entirely by protective clothing. In the case of primary irritants, however, protective gear and thorough cleansing are effective.

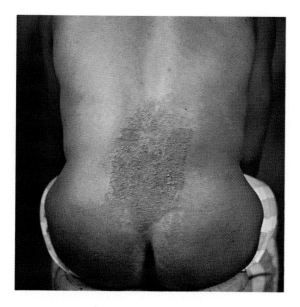

Figure 10-4.   Contact dermatitis from organic mercurial antiseptic

The antiseptic solution was applied prior to obtaining spinal fluid. Mercurial compounds have little place in modern medicine, and the risk of sensitization to them, though low, is hardly worth taking.

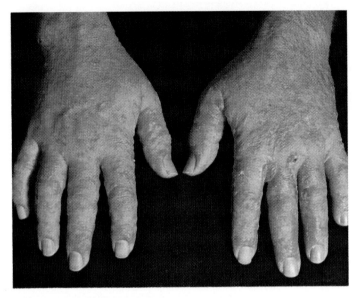

Figure 10–5.   Rhus (poison ivy) dermatitis

The palms of this patient showed little involvement; the thick stratum corneum offers considerable protection.

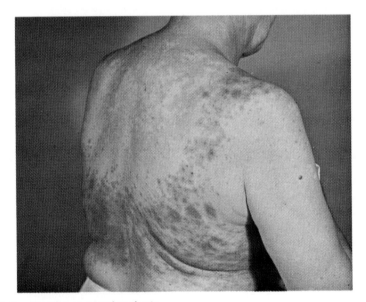

Figure 10–6.   Reaction to Spandex elastic

Unexpected reactions to new items of wearing apparel and to cosmetics often do not come to light until the material is widely distributed and millions of individuals of varying allergic backgrounds come in contact with it.

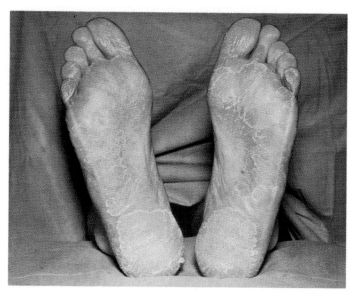

Figure 10–7.   Allergic reaction to shoes

Such reactions are often very difficult to manage. It is important to conduct careful testing to determine the responsible component, i.e., leather, chemical accelerators and additives, dyes, elastic and so forth. Complications resulting from sweating and from secondary infection are common.

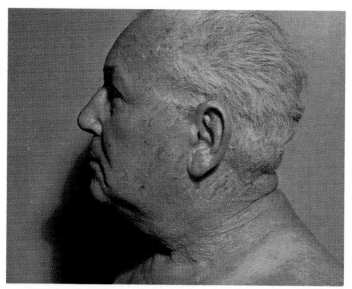

Figure 10–8.   Photoallergic reaction

This patient developed a reactivity to an antiseptic soap containing a brominated salicylanilide, the reaction resulting only when there was the added factor of exposure to sunlight or other ultraviolet sources. Such sensitivity can be extremely persistent; the chemical remains in the skin for prolonged periods.

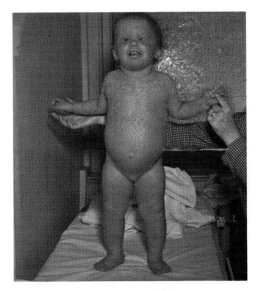

Figure 10–9.   Generalized erythroderma in atopic child

Generalized involvement of this extent is fortunately uncommon in atopic dermatitis. Other syndromes must be considered. Temperature regulation and sweating may be severely compromised.

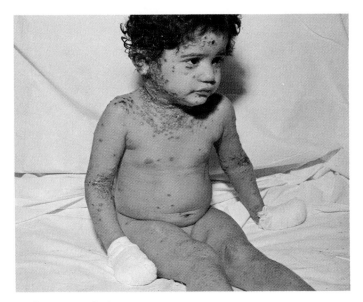

Figure 10–10.   Eczema vaccinatum

This complication developed after vaccination in a child with atopic dermatitis. The systemic reaction was moderate. Note gauze "boxing gloves" to restrict scratching.

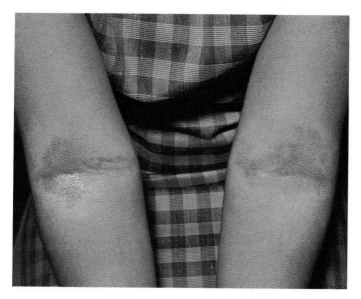

Figure 10–11. Atopic dermatitis

Characteristic antecubital involvement in teen-ager. The itching is often almost unremitting.

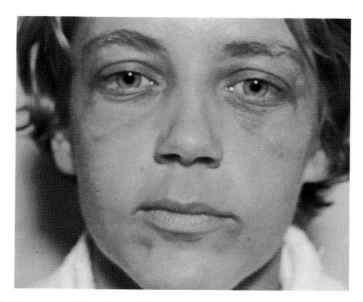

Figure 10–12. Atopic "Mongolian Fold"

This fold below the lower eyelid is characteristic of atopic dermatitis in which there has been involvement of periorbital skin.

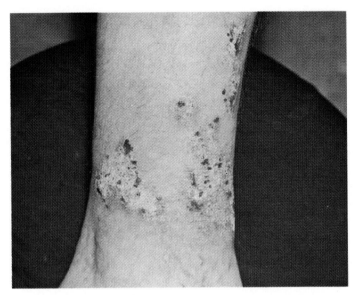

Figure 10–13.   Circumscribed neurodermatitis

Also termed lichen simplex chronicus. Thickening and psoriasiform scaling of the lower leg from repeated scratching. A good example of the self-perpetuating scratch-itch-scratch cycle.

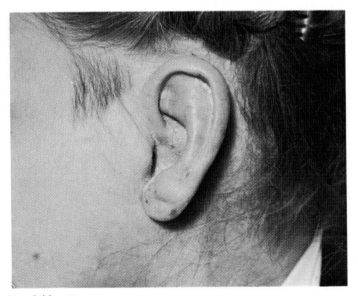

Figure 10–14.   Otitis externa

Chronic scaling and itching of the external ear and auditory canal in a patient with seborrheic scaling of the scalp. A similar picture may be seen in atopic dermatitis and psoriasis.

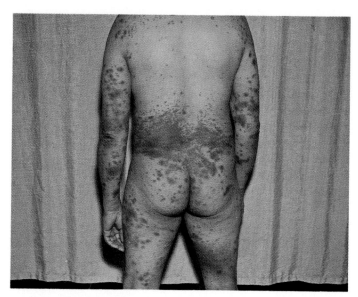

Figure 10–15. Nummular dermatitis

A widespread patchy eruption of initially coin-sized (nummular) inflamed lesions. Seen most frequently in males of middle age or older. May follow a contact dermatitis. A low-grade secondary infection is frequently present.

11

Urticaria and Erythema Multiforme

URTICARIA

The term *urticaria* refers to a solid edema of the skin that may be minimal and evanescent or extensive and chronic. Urticaria may be classified as an anaphylactic syndrome if several organ systems are involved. The lesions of acute urticaria are ordinarily whiter than the normal skin, although there may be a zone of pink erythema surrounding individual lesions. The surface shows follicular indentations (pigskin effect) due to the anchoring effect exerted by hair follicles against the adjacent soft dermal tissue.

In acute urticaria, particularly in a first episode, a precipitating agent ordinarily may be uncovered by careful questioning: an unaccustomed food, a drug, an intercurrent infection, a change in environment or a visitation by a parasite.

As for treatment of mild attacks, nothing is necessary as a rule. Drugs, even antihistamines, offer more risk than benefit unless there is marked itching.

TABLE 11–1 A SUMMARY OF THE ETIOLOGICAL CLASSIFICATION OF URTICARIA*

Allergic Urticaria	
Inhalants	pollens, animal danders, mold spores, feather down, aerosols, smoke, dust and volatile chemicals
Injectants	drugs, diagnostic agents, vaccines, insect stings, serums and blood
Ingestants	drugs, chocolate, eggs, nuts, shellfish, pork, vegetables, coffee, grapes, bananas, strawberries, tomatoes, cow's milk, cheese, wheat, foods derived from yeast fermentation and from mushrooms and occult additive materials found in foods, beverages and medications

*Katz, H. I.: Anaphylactic syndromes. *In* Moschella, S. L., Pillsbury, D. M., and Hurley, H. J.: Dermatology, Vol. I. W. B. Saunders Co., Philadelphia, 1975, p. 229.

TABLE 11–1   A SUMMARY OF THE ETIOLOGICAL CLASSIFICATION
OF URTICARIA (*Continued*)*

Allergic Urticaria (*Continued*)	
Infections	foci of bacterial, fungal, viral and parasitic infections
Contactants	animal products, plant materials, cosmetics, plastic and other chemicals
Drugs	penicillin, aspirin, quinine, sulfonamides, insulin and many others
Exogenous (Obligate) Urticaria due to Urticariogenic Materials	
Aquagenic Chemicals	compound 48/80, Tween 80 and acacia
Drugs	cocaine, morphine, codeine, atropine, quinine, thiamine, pilocarpine, polymyxin B, *d*-tubocurarine, dextran, dehydrocholate sodium (Decholine) and other drugs
Foods	certain citrus fruits, strawberries and certain fish
Toxins	cobra venoms, jellyfish toxin and certain plant and insect toxins
Physical Urticaria	
Dermographic	immediate and delayed
Heat	
Cold	
Light	
Secondary Urticaria	
Infections	infectious mononucleosis, serum hepatitis, malaria, cystitis, sinusitis, prostatitis, cholecystitis, dental abscesses, dermatophytosis, rheumatic fever, trichinosis and other parasitic infections
Collagen vascular diseases	lupus erythematosus, rheumatoid arthritis, dermatomyositis and angiitides
Neoplasia	internal malignancy, lymphoma, and leukemia
Psychogenic	
Other conditions Dermatologic	pemphigoid, dermatitis herpetiformis, amyloidosis, urticaria pigmentosa (mastocytosis) and scabies
Systemic	thyrotoxicosis, hypothyroidism, polycythemia vera, uremic states, pregnancy and serum sickness
Cholinergic Urticaria	
Heat	
Exertion	
Emotional stress	
Pilocarpine	
Acetylcholine	
Hereditary Angioedema	
Autosomal dominant deficiency of alpha-2 globulin inhibitor of C-1 esterase. Originally described by Sir William Osler.	

Chronic recurrent urticaria, especially if the skin lesions are extensive and if there have been signs of respiratory or cardiovascular embarassment, is a much more serious problem. An exhaustive history and general medical survey is always in order.

Urticaria frequently manifests itself by occasional lesions of the skin without systemic signs. Continued observation for precipitating factors is called for. Except when the precipitating factor is an inhalant, scratch and intradermal tests and attempts at hyposensitization are unrewarding in our experience.

Occasional courses of different antihistamines should be tried. Various antihistamines have unpredictable and varying effects, and the side effects of some overshadow their therapeutic benefits. Corticosteroid therapy is generally disappointing in controlling chronic urticaria, and it is not advised!

Patients with chronic urticaria sometimes show variations in the course of their disease, depending on their environment (seasonal, geographic and so on). A specific factor may not be evident to explain the variation.

The importance of salicylates in prolonging chronic urticaria has received increasing emphasis. Shelley (1964) has listed a staggering number of drugs, flavorings, foods, suntan lotions and plants that contain salicylates. Juhlin and associates (1972) have recorded cases of urticaria and asthma due to aspirin-containing food additives.

Prevention and Treatment of Acute Anaphylactic Syndrome

There are few medical events as dramatic as anaphylactic shock. The patient may die within minutes unless proper resuscitation is begun quickly.

The following measures are recommended as guidelines for preventing anaphylaxis.

1. A careful history regarding previous drug reactions, e.g., penicillin or, rarely, sera.

2. Avoidance of administration of penicillin to atopic patients unless absolutely essential.

3. If there is a suggestive history of penicillin sensitivity, the injection should be into the quadriceps or deltoid muscle to allow placement of a tourniquet if it becomes advisable.

Recognition of the following signs of reaction *as early as possible:*

    a. Laryngeal edema, wheezing, hoarseness

    b. Tightness of the chest, cyanosis, hypotension

    c. Cardiovascular collapse, dizziness, loss of consciousness

    d. Loss of sphincter control, convulsive seizures

5. Treatment (See Table 11–2)

TABLE 11–2 TREATMENT OF SYSTEMIC SHOCK STATES*

I. **General Measures**
   A. Start an intravenous infusion of 5 per cent dextrose in water.
   B. Eliminate or reduce absorption of offending material (tourniquet proximal to site of challenge for several minutes, ice application or local epinephrine).
   C. Supine position with clear airway.
   D. Maintain observation for 30 to 60 minutes.
   E. Administer oxygen.
   F. Have resuscitation equipment available.
   G. Observe vital signs.

II. **Generalized Urticaria and Angioedema**
   A. Aqueous epinephrine (0.3 to 0.5 ml., 1:1000 dilution) injection subcutaneously; may be repeated in 15 minutes.
   B. Antihistamine (diphenhydramine [Benadryl] 20 to 50 mg., I.M. or I.V.).

III. **Respiratory Distress**
   A. Aqueous epinephrine as in II-A.
   B. Antihistamine as in II-B.
   C. Maintain airway with intubation or with tracheotomy (surgically or with large bore needle) for severe laryngeal edema.
   D. Aminophylline, 500 mg. in 1000 ml. of 5 per cent dextrose in water given over 1 hour for bronchospasm.

IV. **Cardiovascular Collapse**
   A. Aqueous epinephrine as in II-A or 0.5 to 1.0 ml., 1 to 10,000 dilution, given intravenously or with cardiac needle injected directly into a ventricle in case of cardiac arrest (the latter only as a last resort). External chest wall cardiac massage can be done as a life-saving measure if there is complete cardiac standstill.
   B. Levarterenol bitartrate (Levophed) intravenous infusion—4 ml. of 0.2 per cent solution to 1000 ml. of 5 per cent dextrose in water given 2 ml. per minute for hypotension.
   C. Hydrocortisone hemisuccinate (Solu-cortef) 100 mg. intravenously as a direct push and then an additional 100 mg. given in 1000 ml. of 5 per cent dextrose in water intravenously to reduce late effects from generalized reaction.

*Katz, H. I.: Anaphylactic syndromes. *In* Moschella, S. L., Pillsbury, D. M., and Hurley, H. J.: Dermatology, Vol. I. W. B. Saunders Co., Philadelphia, 1975, p. 237.

ERYTHEMA MULTIFORME

As the term indicates, this syndrome is characterized by considerable variation in the types of lesions it encompasses; it is multiform. It is a symptom complex characterized variably by vivid erythematous, urticarial, bullous and purpuric lesions that appear suddenly in a symmetric distribution.

Although erythema multiforme is regarded as a bullous disease, many cases present no vesicular or bullous lesions. The classic lesion, however, is a round, varicolored, raised bulla. It is seen most commonly on the dorsa of the hands and feet and on the mucous membranes. The typical "target" or "iris" lesion is one of the most pathognomonic in dermatology, although it is not always present. The initial lesions may subside completely, or there may be waves of recurrences. The lesions commonly develop a striking purple coloration. The symptoms of erythema multiforme are generally moderate, although there may be notable exceptions in the bullous types, especially the Stevens-Johnson syndrome.

A striking feature of erythema multiforme is the frequency with which an attack is preceded by a lesion of herpes simplex — possibly half of all cases in our experience. The mechanism involved has not yet been determined. Other factors have been reported as preceding erythema multiforme, such as systemic infections, various drugs, deep x-ray therapy and malignancy. We have observed a number of cases of the latter. In some instances, resection of the malignant growth is followed by resolution of the skin lesions.

Treatment

The type and intensity of treatment needed to control erythema multiforme depends upon the severity of the reaction and, in some cases, on the etiology. Mild disease may not require treatment. More extensive lesions may be controlled with topical steroid preparations and bland shake lotions. Extensive erosive and bullous disease, on the other hand, will require hospitalization, topical treatment similar to that used for extensive burns, and immunosuppressive doses of systemic corticosteroids. In each variation of the disease, an intense effort should be made to determine the etiologic factors of the reaction, to remove them and to prevent secondary complications of the disease and treatment. Nonessential drugs should be discontinued or group substitutions made. Every precaution should be taken to minimize the risks of bacterial, viral, yeast and fungal superinfection, particularly in the immunosuppressed patient.

Erythema multiforme includes serious bullous types, which may be fatal. The best example of this is the Stevens-Johnson syndrome (originally termed ectodermosis erosiva pluriorificialis). Children and young adults are most frequently affected. The initial picture is alarming. Conjunctivitis, rhinitis, stomatitis, urethritis and balanitis appear suddenly. Within a few days, widespread bullous, erosive and papular lesions develop. Toxicity is severe. The eye complications are especially grave. Prompt corticosteroid therapy in large immunosuppressive doses is indicated initially. Topical treatment is similar to that used for an extensive burn. The etiologic factors cannot be precisely determined in most cases. The mortality rate is on the order of 20 to 25 per cent.

ERYTHEMA PERSTANS

This is an all-encompassing term for a variety of annular and circinate recurrent skin lesions of generally unknown etiology. One of the original designations was Darier's erythema annulare centrifugum, and through the years perhaps a dozen more or less obscure alternatives have been used. Most have been discarded.

Erythema perstans is found chiefly on the trunk and thighs. The primary lesion is a slightly inflamed, annular papule that enlarges in rather spectacular fashion. New lesions develop, sometimes within the old one. There may be some scaling of the borders. Moderate pruritis is sometimes noted.

Patients with erythema perstans deserve careful study, including biopsy of the lesion and survey for hematologic or solid tumor malignancy. There may be a sensitivity to microbiologic organisms, and a therapeutic trial of griseofulvin and nystatin is worthwhile. Local therapy is ineffective, and systemic corticosteroid therapy — at least in prolonged courses — is not justified.

REFERENCES

Juhlin, L., Michaëlsson, G., and Zetterström, O.: Urticaria and asthma induced by food and drug additives in patients with aspirin hypersensitivity. J. Allergy Clin. Immunol. 50:92–8, 1972.

Shelley, W. B.: Birch pollen and aspirin psoriasis. A study in salicylate hypersensitivity. J.A.M.A. 189:985–8, 1964.

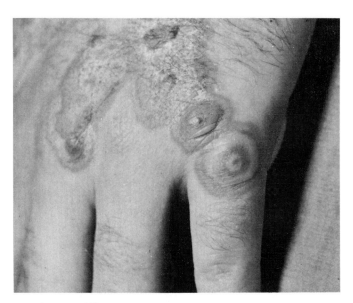

Figure 11–1.   Erythema multiforme

The macules, papules, vesicles, bullae and target or iris lesions seen here typify the multiple forms taken by lesions of this disorder. This patient's disease was preceded by an episode of "fever blisters."

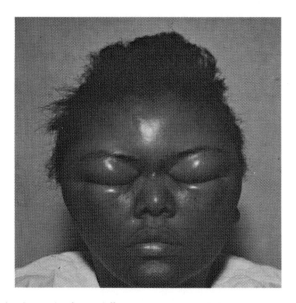

Figure 11–2.   Urticaria (angioedema) following ingestion of fish

The possibility of obstructive laryngeal edema or anaphylactoid shock must be kept in mind with a reaction of this severity.

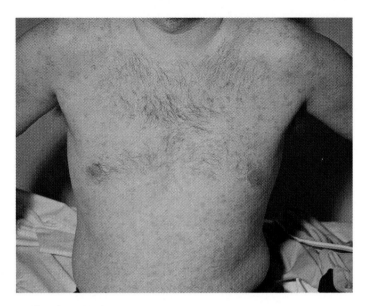

Figure 11–3. Chronic urticaria

Pinkish lesions, many annular, occurring regularly in showers. Urticaria is sometimes periodic, with lesions tending to occur at certain times of the day or night. Antihistaminic and corticosteroid therapy were indifferently effective in this patient.

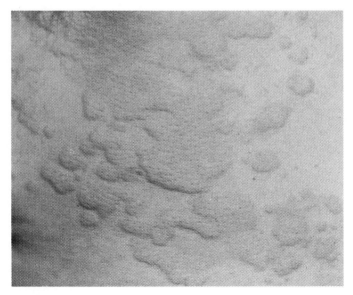

Figure 11–4. Urticaria

Edematous lesions with typical pigskin appearance caused by follicular restraint on the swelling. Patients with urticaria frequently have bouts of varying severity, from a few small lesions to marked angioedema.

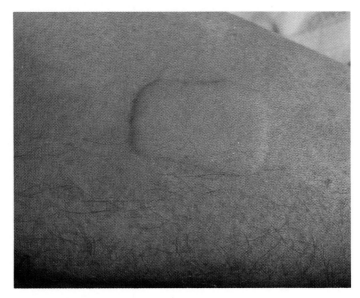

Figure 11–5. Cold urticaria

This lesion was produced by contact with a container filled with ice water. Such sensitivity may be so marked as to require residence in a warm climate. The patient also had chronic leukemia. Bathing in cold water may produce severe histamine shock.

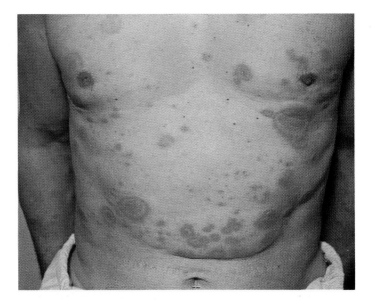

Figure 11–6. Chronic erythema multiforme

This patient sustained repeated showers of ringed erythematous urticarial lesions which evolved more slowly than in erythema multiforme. Probably to be classified in the erythema perstans group, which has a formidable alternate terminology. Often extremely chronic. Specific cause usually not determinable.

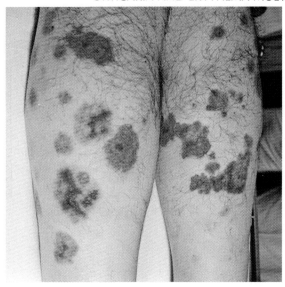

Figure 11–7.   Purpuric erythema multiforme

As the term "multiforme" indicates, the syndrome may vary considerably in appearance. In this patient the initial lesions were largely bullous, with purpura developing later. Hematologic study obviously indicated.

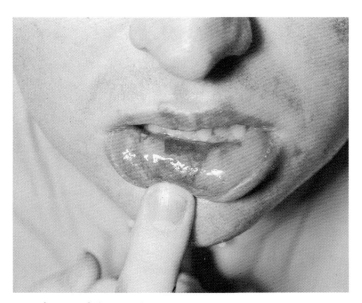

Figure 11–8.   Erythema multiforme of lip

Typical oral erosive lesion. This patient had sustained repeated attacks, usually in the spring and ordinarily preceded by herpes simplex.

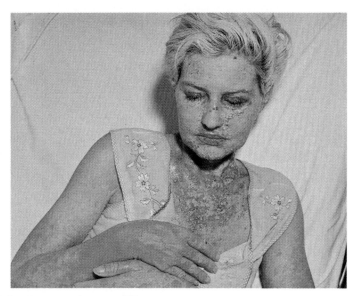

Figure 11-9.   Severe erythema multiforme

Because this variant was assigned such a long name originally, it has become known as the Stevens-Johnson syndrome. The cutaneous, conjunctival and orificial involvement are severe. May be fatal, especially in children.

Bullous Diseases

12

The formation of large vesicles and bullae in the skin or oral cavity, particularly if recurrent, represents a tissue insult that demands classification as promptly as possible. Bullae may signal passing disorders or the onset of very chronic diseases having significant morbidity and mortality. Pustular variants are common and most of these diseases are susceptible to secondary bacterial infection. This group of diseases varies from very common to rare.

COMMON

Physical factors—mechanical rubbing, heat, cold
Sunlight—overexposure, drug-induced photosensitivity or toxicity, porphyria

Reactions to systemically administered drugs
Infections—bacterial, fungal, viral
Contact dermatitis
Erythema multiforme

UNCOMMON

Pemphigus vulgaris
Pemphigus vegetans
Epidermolysis bullosa
"Benign" mucosal pemphigoid
Dermatitis herpetiformis

Bullous lichen planus
Toxic epidermal necrolysis
Diphtheria cutis
Chronic benign familial pemphigus
Pemphigus erythematosus

The common bullous diseases are largely dealt with elsewhere in this volume, and this section is concerned principally with the relatively uncommon ones, all of which have significant systemic medical implications.

PEMPHIGUS VULGARIS

This is a classic bullous disease, one that will rarely be seen in general practice. The treatment available in large medical centers is required for care of patients with this extremely chronic disease. Careful monitoring of the toxic effects of the corticosteroid and immunosuppressive drugs essential for the proper management of pemphigus vulgaris and frequent evaluations of the patient's progress are necessary. *Early diagnosis and vigorous, prompt treatment are essential to the control, if not the cure, of pemphigus.*

The primary lesion of pemphigus is a vesicle or bulla. The most common initial site of involvement is the mouth, where the bullae quickly rupture to form painful erosions. The painful oral and pharyngeal lesions soon interfere with eating, drinking and talking. On the skin, lesions often arise on what appears to be normal skin, principally in the "seborrheic" areas. Low-grade, mixed superficial infection occurs, and the affected areas may emit a disagreeable "mousy" odor. An acute cellulitis does not occur. The nursing care of patients with extensive pemphigus requires devotion and skill.

Pemphigus occurs most commonly, but by no means exclusively, in persons of Jewish descent. It is principally a disease of middle age but may occur toward the end of life's spectrum.

The primary clinical laboratory procedure of use in establishing a diagnosis of pemphigus is the Tzanck test. Smears taken from the base of a bulla and stained with Giemsa stain demonstrate a typical acantholysis (loss of intercellular bridges) in the lower epidermis. This finding, in connection with the clinical picture, is highly suggestive, though not diagnostically conclusive. The histopathologic picture is usually strongly suggestive of the correct diagnosis. Confirmation of the diagnosis may usually be accomplished through the use of direct and indirect immunofluorescent tissue staining techniques (Table 12–1).

If the evidence for pemphigus is strong, referral of the patient to an experienced "pemphigus center" is advised. The prospective rapid downhill course of pemphigus in terms of infection, "toxemia" and disturbances in serum proteins and electrolytes is so ominous as to demand complete evaluation and appropriate management as promptly and expertly as possible.

Pemphigus takes other forms, but these are so rare as to be of minimal concern in general practice. Briefly, they are as follows:

Pemphigus Vegetans.   As the term indicates, this variant tends to develop verrucoid vegetations at sites of pemphigus on the face and in interdigital areas of the axillae and anogenital region. Oral lesions occur. The early histologic changes are similar to those of pemphigus vulgaris but later become more exuberant and proliferative.

Pemphigus Erythematosus.   This variant morphologically suggests a combination of lupus erythematosus and seborrheic dermatitis, affecting the scalp, malar prominences and upper trunk. The general health of the patient is usually unaffected, and the prognosis is better than in other forms of pemphigus.

Pemphigus Foliaceus.   This variant is a relatively mild disease that occurs principally in older persons. It may be related to the Brazilian pemphigus fogo selvagem, a possibly endemic viral infection, with which the authors have had no personal experience.

Treatment

Before the advent of corticosteroid therapy, the mortality rate approached 100 per cent following a disease course of from several months to over a year. Pemphigus per se does not become systemic, but death results variously from infection, hypoproteinemia, electrolyte imbalance, starvation and reactions to treatment.

Because of the vigorous treatment employed for pemphigus vulgaris, it is especially necessary that the diagnosis be certain. Treatment should be initiated decisively, not tentatively. An initial dose of prednisone of 80 to 120 mg. per day is recommended. Improvement will ordinarily become evident within a week or two, and gradual reduction of the dose may then be undertaken. As the dose of prednisone is reduced, alternate-day administration should be attempted. If the pemphigus has not responded to corticosteroids, addition of an immunosuppressive agent may be advisable — usually methotrexate in an initial dose of 25 mg. by mouth weekly. Other immunosuppressive agents, such as azathioprine and cyclophosphamide, may also be used, but such therapy is potentially very toxic and should not be employed by those inexperienced in chemotherapy.

The topical therapy of pemphigus does not affect the course of the disease but may ease discomfort and combat odor. An ordinary shake lotion is helpful, as is a thorough talc powdering of the bed sheets. Saline, manganese oxide (MnO_4) or oatmeal baths are helpful. Watch should be kept for evidence of secondary infection. Cultures ordinarily show a highly mixed flora.

DERMATITIS HERPETIFORMIS (Duhring's Disease)

Dermatitis herpetiformis is an extremely chronic vesicular disease characterized by suddenly erupting groups of small vesicles distributed over the forearms, scapular area, sacral area, buttocks and thighs. Itching is intense, and scratching soon obliterates the vesicles.

Direct immunofluorescent staining of the basement membrane demonstrates the presence of large quantities of IgA. Smaller quantities of IgG and complement are also present. There is no intercellular or basement membrane fluorescence on indirect immunofluorescence (Table 12–1).

TABLE 12–1 IMMUNOFLUORESCENCE STAINING PATTERN IN AUTOIMMUNE DISEASES OF THE SKIN, ILLUSTRATING DEMONSTRATION OF IMMUNOGLOBULINS (Ig) AND COMPLEMENT (C)†

Disease	Direct Intercellular		Direct Basement Membrane				Indirect Inter-cellular	Indirect Base-ment Mem-brane
	IgG	*C*	*IgG*	*IgA*	*IgM*	*C*		
Dermatitis herpetiformis	–	–	+	++++	0	+	0	0
Lupus erythematosus								
Systemic lupus (SLE)*	–	–	++++	+	+	+	0	0
Discoid lupus**	–	–	++++	+	+	+	0	0
Bullous pemphigoid	–	–	++++	+	+	+	0	+
Pemphigus vulgaris	++++	+	–	–	–	–	+	0

*involved and uninvolved skin
**uninvolved skin only
†From Bellanti, J. A.: Immunology II, W. B. Saunders Co., Philadelphia, 1978, p. 611.

A curious gastrointestinal accompaniment of dermatitis herpetiformis in some two-thirds of patients is an enteropathy similar to that seen in celiac disease. Stockbrugger and associates (1976) have recently described achlorhydria, atrophic gastritis and elevated levels of antibodies against parietal cells. Shuster and associates (1968) reported variable results from treatment with a gluten-free diet.

Treatment

A long-used "specific" for dermatitis herpetiformis is sulfapyridine, given in a dose of 2 gm. per day. With improvement, which is fairly constant, the dose is reduced to 0.5 gm. to 1 gm. per day. Unfortunately, sulfapyridine is productive of a variety of reactions, ranging from headaches, gastrointestinal upset, hematologic abnormalities and renal stones to psychic disturbances and dermatologic reactions that sometimes require discontinuance of the drug. Readministration in small doses is sometimes possible, depending on the significance of the original reaction. Fortunately, an effective alternate treatment, diaminodiphenylsulfone (DDS, dapsone) is also effective, though not without significant toxic effects. The initial dose of DDS is 200 to 300 mg. per day with reduction to a range of 50 to 100 mg. per day as soon as possible. The most important side effects of DDS are an anemia resulting from delayed red cell survival, hemolysis and methemoglobulinemia, all of which are dose-related.

Corticosteroid therapy is a much less desirable alternative therapy in dermatitis herpetiformis. Unfortunately, because of the extreme chronicity and maddening pruritis of the disease, prolonged treatment is necessary, thus accentuating the toxic effect of any form of systemic treatment.

BULLOUS PEMPHIGOID

Bullous pemphigoid is a chronic blistering disease that differs from pemphigus vulgaris in several respects, although initial differentiation may be difficult. The disease is characterized by tense bullae that may arise from skin of normal appearance or from erythematous skin. The lesions tend to occur principally on the lower abdomen, groin, inner aspects of the thighs and flexor surfaces of the forearms. Age of onset is usually above 50 — greater than in pemphigus vulgaris. There is no racial or ethnic predisposition to the disease. Microscopically there is no acantholysis, as is seen in pemphigus, and immunofluorescence is observed at the basement membrane rather than intercellularly. Itching is a prominent feature in some patients, and the general discomfort is extreme.

Treatment

Systemic corticosteroid therapy is indicated in extensive cases, but the dose should not be as high as is required in pemphigus. Every effort should be made to reduce the steroid dose — sometimes by the addition of methotrexate. For localized lesions, topical corticosteroid therapy may suffice. The disease persists for months or years and is sometimes fatal.

EPIDERMOLYSIS BULLOSA

This uncommon disease is characterized by the development of bullae at sites of minor trauma. Various classifications have been proposed on the basis of genetic, histopathologic and electron microscopic studies, but a purely clinical approach will suffice for this summary.

Epidermolysis Bullosa Simplex. Bullae develop within the first year of life on sites of trauma, such as the elbows, knees, hands and feet. They heal without scarring, unless infected.

Dystrophic Epidermolysis Bullosa. This disease usually becomes evident in early infancy and includes dystrophic changes, resulting in fusion and severe deformity of the fingers and toes, as well as severe scarring at other sites of trauma.

Epidermolysis Bullosa Letalis. This is a severe blistering disease that is ordinarily fatal within the first 2 years of life.

Treatment

There is no satisfactory treatment for epidermolysis bullosa. Every effort should be made to combat trauma to the skin. For example, the patient should wear fleece-lined slippers and protective gloves when practical. Evidence of infection can be treated with an antibiotic ointment or, if indicated, systemic antibiotics.

TOXIC EPIDERMAL NECROLYSIS

This disease, which affects young children and adults alike, is a toxic erythema in which the skin undergoes epidermal necrosis and peeling, resulting in the common designation of "scalded skin syndrome." The microscopic pictures in the pediatric and adult forms differ somewhat, but the course of the disease is similar. A considerable variety of etiologic factors has been proposed, including infection, especially Group II phage type 71 staphylococci, and numerous drugs.

Topical management is similar to that given for burns. Corticosteroids given in immunosuppressive doses are useful — often life saving — in cases of drug-induced toxic epidermal necrolysis but are of little value in bacterially induced disease. Penicillinase-resistant penicillin is the drug of choice in staphylococcus-induced disease. Even with the best of care and early appropriate drug therapy, the mortality rate is on the order of 25 per cent.

REFERENCES

Shuster, S., Watson, A. J., and Marks, J.: Coeliac syndrome in dermatitis herpitiformis. Lancet 1:1101–6, 1968.
Stockbrügger, R., Andersson, H., Gillberg, R., et al.: Auto-immune atrophic gastritis in patient with dermatitis herpetiformis. Acta Derm. Venereol. (Stockholm) 56(2):111–113, 1976.

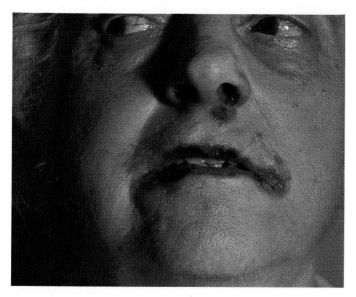

Figure 12–1. Pemphigus vulgaris

Oral and nasal mucous membrane involvement. The oral lesions frequently make eating extremely difficult and the nutritional problem may become very significant.

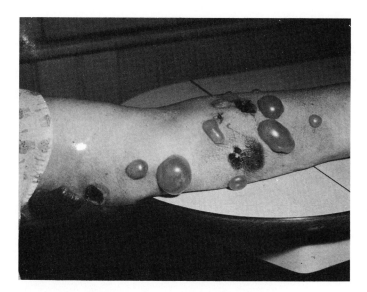

Figure 12–2. Bullous pemphigoid

Tense bullae on a nonerythematous base are typical. Hemorrhage develops in older lesions. A search for an internal malignancy often is rewarding in older patients.

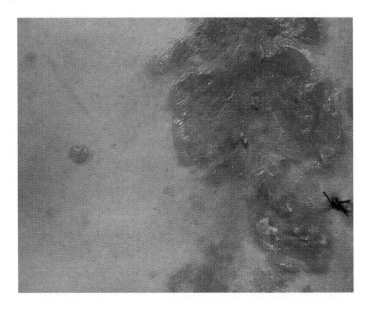

Figure 12–3.   Pemphigus of the back

Typical bullous and eroded lesions. As seen in smaller lesion on left, new bullae develop in what appears to be normal skin. Pemphigus of this severity is very susceptible to infection, and in extensive involvement, the serous protein losses may be significant.

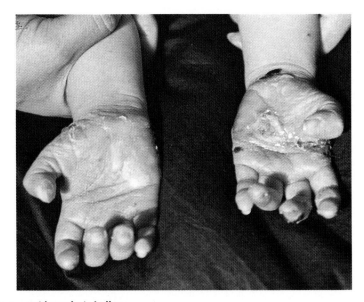

Figure 12–4.   Epidermolysis bullosa

A genetically endowed tendency to react to ordinary day-to-day trauma with formation of bullae. There are two types, one comparatively mild with minor destructive characteristics, the other extremely destructive of underlying tissue and bone.

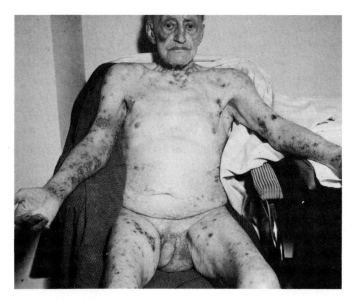

Figure 12–5. Dermatitis herpetiformis

Intense itching and vigorous scratching resulted in the many open erosions on this patient's skin. Sulfones brought dramatic relief.

13 | Cutaneous Manifestations of Systemic Disease

A very diverse group of systemic diseases may be associated with lesions of the skin. The more common of these are discussed in other chapters of this volume. There remains, however, a considerble group in which the alerting diagnostic sign is cutaneous. Some of them are summarized briefly herewith. This pictorial series of reminders is by no means complete, but it includes a number of distinctive syndromes, varying from fairly common to rare. Most of them are compelling indications for further study.

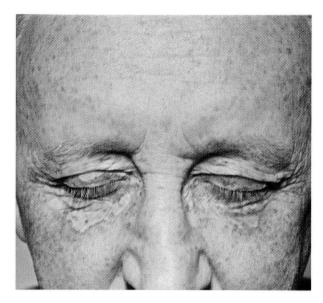

Figure 13–1.   Xanthelasma

Soft plaques of xanthoma involving the eyelids and circumocular skin. These lesions were long in developing to their full extent. Thoroughgoing study of lipid metabolism and cardiovascular status is indicated.

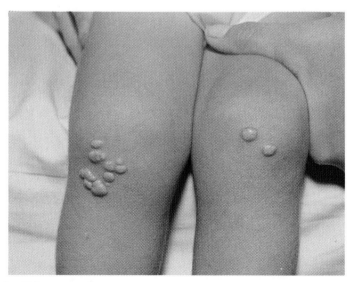

Figure 13–2.   Tuberous xanthoma

Characteristic nodular xanthomatous lesion over the knees. Other areas that may be involved are the elbows, skin folds of the palms, the buttocks, back of the heel, tendons and ligaments. General medical study essential.

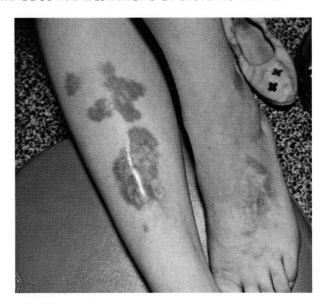

Figure 13–3.   Necrobiosis lipoidica

A clinically very characteristic lesion occurring principally on the pretibial surfaces, in diabetic or prediabetic patients. Ulceration sometimes occurs, particularly after biopsy. May respond to topical or intralesional corticosteroids.

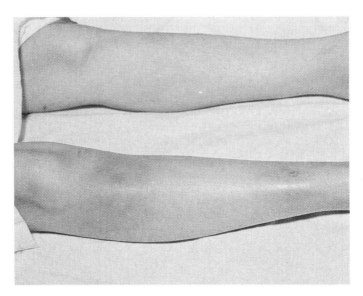

Figure 13–4.   Erythema nodosum

Inflamed nodules and plaques, most commonly on the anterior legs. Streptococcal infection is the most common excitant, but many other infections may induce this sensitization syndrome. It is seen most frequently in young female adults. Drugs, particularly the birth control pill, are also common initiating agents. Sarcoidosis should also be considered.

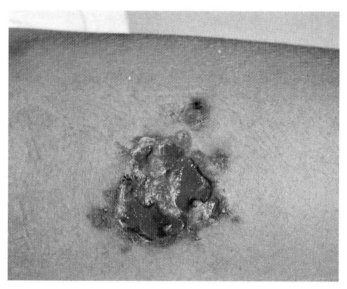

Figure 13–5. Sporotrichosis

A highly characteristic deep fungal infection. Rapidly developing ulcer with satellite lesions. Induration of and nodules along the draining lymphatics. Rapid response to modest doses of potassium iodide.

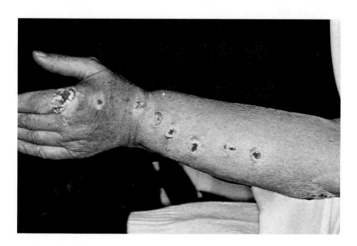

Figure 13–6. Sporotrichosis

Sporothrix schenckii inoculation occurred at the base of the index finger. The development of ulcero-nodular lesions along the course of a lymphatic is characteristic.

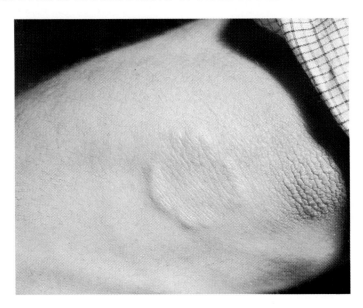

Figure 13–7.   Granuloma annulare

A suspicion-arousing but completely benign lesion, without systemic significance, except, rarely, diabetes. Characteristic picture on biopsy. Lesions may come and go for years. May respond to soft irradiation or intralesional corticosteroid therapy.

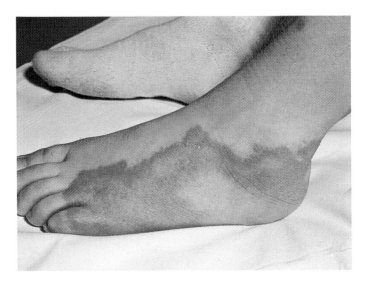

Figure 13–8.   Tuberculoid leprosy

Involvement of the foot, along with the arms and face, in a ten-year-old Greek boy who had been brought to the U.S.A. two years previously. His mother was found to have lepromatous leprosy, undoubtedly the source of the boy's infection. He was noninfectious. The response to dapsone (4-4'diaminodiphenylsulphone, DDS) therapy was very satisfactory. (Raque, C. J., and Thew, M. A.: Atypical erythema nodosum in an immigrant. A clue to two cases of leprosy. Cutis 6:395–400, 1970.)

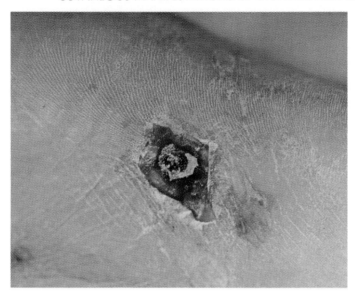

Figure 13-9. Diphtheria cutis

Typical ulcer with adherent brownish-black eschar. Local anesthesia is characteristic. Encountered with some frequency during World War II in southwest Pacific and China-Burma-India theaters, less frequently in European and Mediterranean theaters. The exotoxins from skin lesions may produce the same cardiac and neurologic complications seen in pharyngeal diphtheria. (Pictorial Service, U.S. Army Medical Department, Dr. Clarence S. Livingood.)

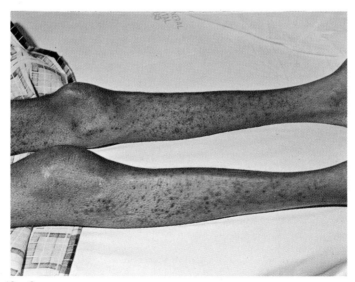

Figure 13-10. Scurvy

The perifollicular purpuric lesions in avitaminosis-C are almost pathognomonic. Sometimes called "bachelor's disease" — too little fresh vitamin C food and too much alcohol.

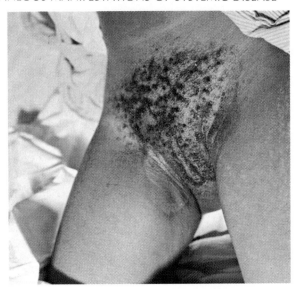

Figure 13–11. Pellagra

The resemblance to tinea cruris or erythrasma is obvious; in fact, such organisms may be present, though not demonstrable in this patient. Other signs of pellagra were present.

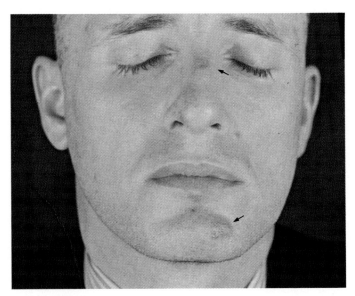

Figure 13–12. Sarcoidosis

Two small facial lesions. The biopsy picture is characteristic and in some patients may be the only means by which the diagnosis may be made with certainty.

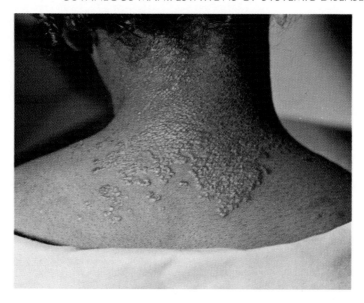

Figure 13–13.   Sarcoidosis

Multiple coalescent papular lesions. They may regress and recur for no apparent reason. Not all patients with sarcoidosis have skin lesions. Those that do often have significant systemic disease.

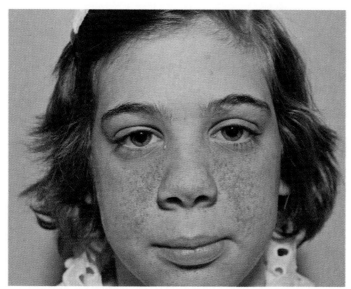

Figure 13–14.   Adenoma sebaceum

Characteristic distribution of small whitish or reddish papules associated with tuberous sclerosis of the brain and, frequently, with mental deficiency and epilepsy.

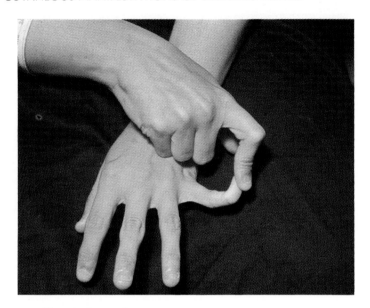

Figure 13–15.   Ehlers-Danlos syndrome

Hyperextensibility of joints associated with hyperelasticity of skin (cutis laxa) and scarring after slight injury.

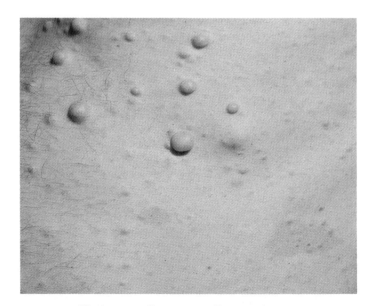

Figure 13–16.   von Recklinghausen's disease (neurofibromatosis)

Characteristic combination of brown flat pigmented areas (café au lait spots) and soft tumors arising on peripheral nerves. The pigmented areas are present at birth or appear in early childhood; the nodules not until after puberty. Tumors may develop on any somatic, cranial or autonomic nerve. Up to 10 per cent of the patients may develop pheochromocytomas.

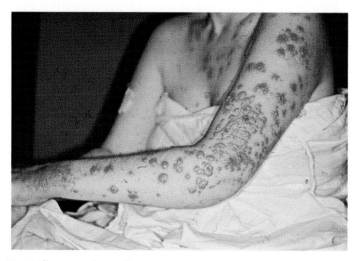

Figure 13–17.   Bullous eruption and cancer

This extensive erythema multiforme-like eruption occurred in a patient with gastric adenocarcinoma. The relation of the skin lesions to the internal tumor is sometimes established by the disappearance of the lesion if the tumor is completely resected.

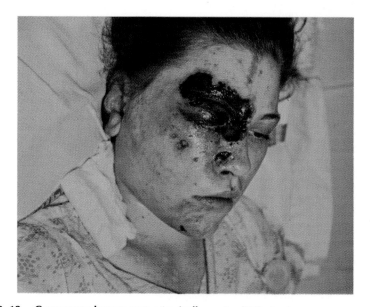

Figure 13–18.   Gangrenous herpes zoster (varicella–zoster [VZ] virus)

In patient with uncontrolled juvenile diabetes. Gangrenous zoster is almost certain to have as a background a specific disease or general debilitation.

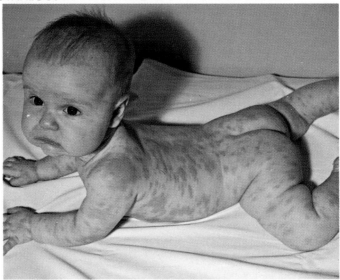

Figure 13–19. Mastocytosis (urticaria pigmentosa)

Extensive nodules and plaques of mast cells in infant. The lesions urticate when rubbed, due to release of histamine. There is no satisfactory treatment, but the outlook is for eventual involution.

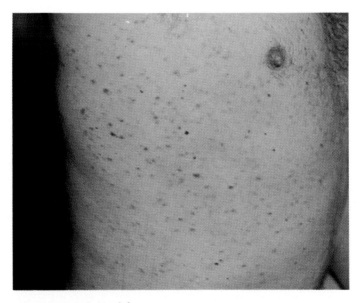

Figure 13–20. Mastocytosis in adult

Unlike the course in children, urticaria pigmentosa does not involute in adults, and extensive involvement of liver, spleen, bone marrow and other organs may occur.

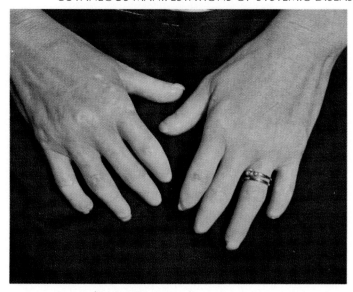

Figure 13–21. Systemic sclerosis (scleroderma)

Induration, whiteness and stiffness of finger (sclerodactylia) with tendency to chronic dry ulcers at points of trauma. Associated calcinosis is not uncommon. A history of preceding Raynaud's phenomenon is almost always obtainable.

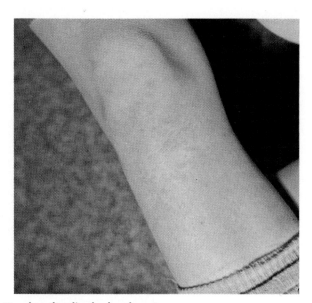

Figure 13–22. Morphea (localized scleroderma)

White indurated sclerotic areas which may extend over a period of months or years, sometimes in linear fashion. Systemic involvement unlikely.

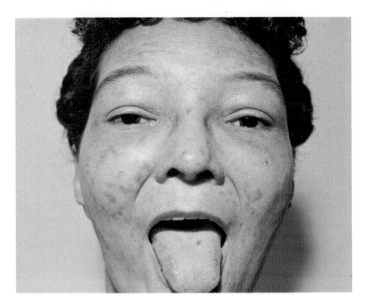

Figure 13–23. Scleroderma

Pigmentary changes and telangiectasia in early systemic sclerosis. The tongue was somewhat thickened and indurated.

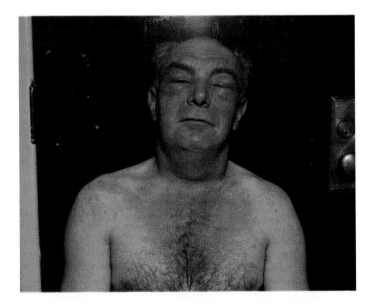

Figure 13–24. Dermatomyositis

Florid "heliotrope" erythema that may be mistaken for a contact dermatitis or photosensitivity. There are characteristic scaling patches at the base of the fingernails and on the knuckles and backs of the fingers. In adults, an underlying malignancy occurs with considerable frequency.

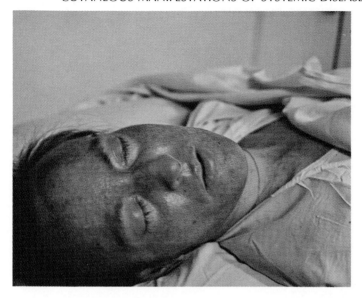

Figure 13–25.   Acute systemic lupus erythematosus

A suffused dusky erythema with telangiectatic spots and diffuse hair loss. The patient expired a short time later of renal failure.

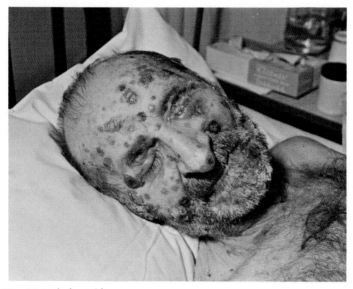

Figure 13–26.   Mycosis fungoides

Terminal tumor stage of this lymphoma.

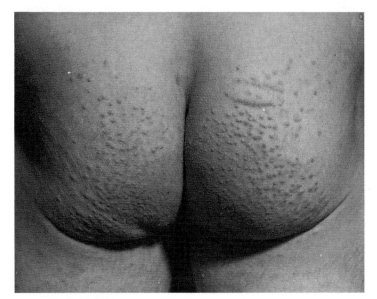

Figure 13–27.   Eruptive xanthoma

Suddenly appearing papular yellow to red lesions in patient with hyperlipemia and hypercholesteremia, related to underlying systemic disease, in this case poorly controlled diabetes mellitus. Hepatic and renal disease may be factors.

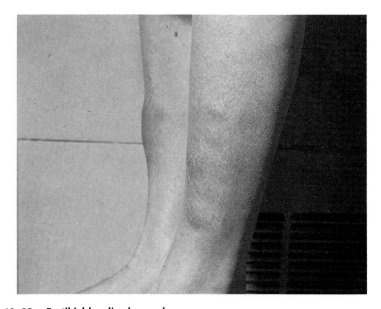

Figure 13–28.   Pretibial localized myxedema

Mucinous infiltrates occurring in association with hyperthyroidism. The prominence of the lesions may be diminished by topical corticosteroid creams with occlusion or by intralesional steroid injections.

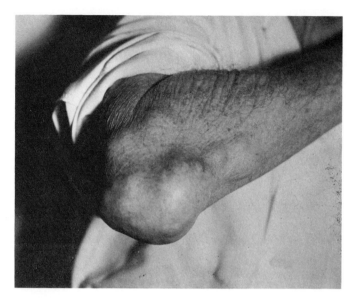

Figure 13–29. Gout

The tophi seen in this patient with gouty arthritis must be distinguished from xanthomas, rheumatoid nodules, ganglions, calcinosis cutis and calcified cysts.

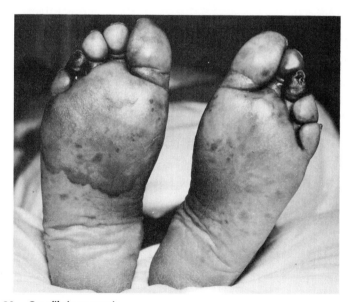

Figure 13–30. Cryofibrinogenemia

Primary and secondary cryofibrinogenemia are described. Cold sensitivity with or without gangrene of digits is the most common clinical complaint. Underlying malignancies of the lung, stomach, ovaries and prostate are common. Chronic lymphatic leukemia, fibrosarcomas and acute rheumatic fever have also been associated with the abnormality.

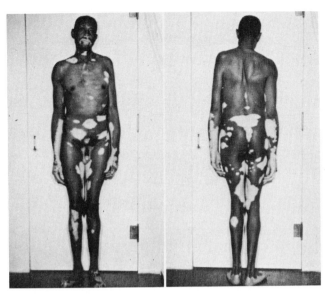

Figure 13–31.   Vitiligo

This acquired patchy, macular, symmetrical, chronic depigmentation of the skin, found most commonly about body orifices, and intertriginous areas, over bony prominences and on exposed surfaces, may have its onset in childhood; but occurs most frequently in young adults. It is probably an autoimmune disease. It is frequently associated with adult-onset diabetes mellitus and may be associated with hyperthyroidism, hypothyroidism, pernicious anemia, hypoparathyroidism, Addison's disease, alopecia areata and the collagen diseases. Less frequently, it has been associated with atopic eczema, psoriasis, malignant melanoma, gastric carcinoma, IgA deficiency and a variety of oculocutaneous syndromes. Therapy is not very satisfactory. Topical and systemic psoralens combined with sunlight or ultraviolet light-A are of limited value. Stains produce inconsistent cosmetic results. The same can be said for topical and intralesional corticosteroids.

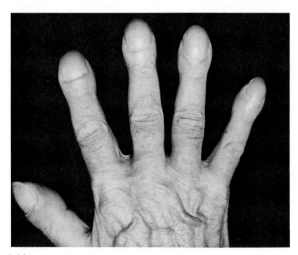

Figure 13–32.   Clubbing

An increase in the curvature of the nail plate laterally and longitudinally, combined with the loss of the normal angle between the nail plate and the proximal nail fold, is a physical characteristic that may be an autosomal dominant familial characteristic, part of extensive malformation syndromes or acquired. Acquired clubbing is most frequently seen with cardiopulmonary disease, particularly bronchogenic carcinoma, bronchiectesis, emphysema and extensive pulmonary tuberculosis. Involution of the clubbing may follow successful treatment of the underlying disease process.

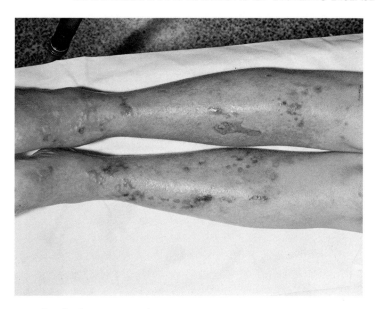

Figure 13–33. Porphyria cutanea tarda (PCT)

An acquired disease of adulthood, PCT most commonly manifests itself as a photosensitivity. Hyperpigmentation, skin fragility with blistering, milia, scarring, sclerodermoid skin changes and hypertrichosis fully characterize the clinical manifestations. The elevated excretion of urinary uroporphyrin and coproporphyrin, combined with increased fecal coproporphyrin and protoporphyrin, completes the syndrome. Serial phlebotomy and low dose chloroquine therapy will produce improvement of clinical and laboratory signs of the disease.

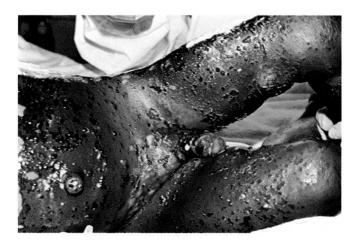

Figure 13–34. Toxic epidermal necrolysis

This child had a group II phage-type 71 staphylococcal pneumonitis. Bullae were intraepithelial, distinguishing it from the drug-induced lesions that are subepidermal. Specific antibiotic—not corticosteroid—therapy is indicated in the staphylococcal-induced disease. Steroid therapy may be useful in the drug-induced disease.

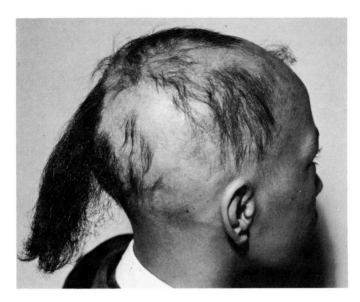

Figure 13–35. Alopecia areata

Sudden onset of a rapid nonscarring loss of hair typifies this disease. Local or disseminated patchy loss of hair, with or without vertical and horizontal pitting of the nails, may occur. Total loss of scalp hair may occur, and rarely, universal alopecia. Vitiligo, lupus erythematosus, thyroiditis and other autoimmune diseases seem to have an increased association with alopecia areata. Recovery is often spontaneous if the initial hair loss is limited. The prognosis for regrowth is poor if extensive hair loss occurs. The beneficial effects of topical and intralesional corticosteroids are usually only temporary. It is probably an autoimmune disease.

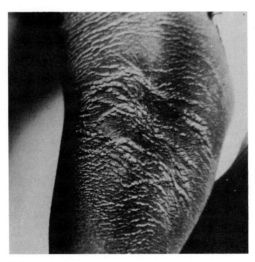

Figure 13–36. Acanthosis nigricans

Gastrointestinal pain, tarry stools, and weight loss preceded the sudden onset of this eruption. At laparotomy a gastric carcinoma was demonstrated. Similar skin lesions are occasionally seen in endocrinopathies and exogenous obesity.

Reactions to Light and Other Environmental Stresses

PHOTOSENSITIVITY REACTIONS*

Of all the ubiquitous physical and chemical forces in man's environment, sunlight produces the widest variety of changes in the skin, both acute and chronic. The chronic changes of accelerated aging and subsequent epitheliomas are commonplace. In recent decades an increasing number of systemically or topically administered chemicals have been shown to have phototoxic or photoallergic potential. The morphologic patterns of acute reactions to sunlight are varied and are designated by a considerable variety of names,** depending on appearance and associated systemic disease.

Certain individuals are endowed at birth with disturbances that make them unusually sensitive to sunlight. Of these, two rare but serious conditions deserve mention. In xeroderma pigmentosum the affected child responds to sunlight with the development of keratoses and prickle cell epitheliomas that are ordinarily lethal in time. In other children, a peculiar and distinctive disturbance of porphyrin metabolism erythropoietic protoporphyria, renders them unduly sensitive. The only individuals who are completely protected from the chronic effects of overexposure to sunlight are dark-skinned blacks. With descending degrees of pigmentation the risks of chronic exposure increase. Blondes and rufous-skinned individuals (red heads), especially the latter, are almost always destined to premature aging and eventual epitheliomas if they persist in chronic overexposure to sunlight. It is never too early in life to impress on these individuals the necessity of avoiding repeated reactions. Epitheliomas are very uncommon in blacks.

---

*We are indebted to Isaac Willis, M.D., of the Department of Dermatology, Emory University School of Medicine, for suggestions and investigative data.
**Examples are actinic erythema multiforme, hydroa aestivale, xeroderma pigmentosum, pellagra, erythropoietic protoporphyria, porphyria cutanea tarda, lupus erythematosus, drug-induced photosensitivity, polymorphic light eruption, hydroa vacciniforme.

The range of skin and systemic diseases associated with increased sensitivity to sunlight is large (Table 14–1). Among these are porphyria cutanea tarda and pellagra, the latter fortunately uncommon in well-nourished populations. Discoid lupus erythematosus is variably light-sensitive, some individuals not showing any such tendency, while a high proportion of patients with frank systemic lupus are sensitive. A reaction beginning in the skin may exacerbate the entire systemic disease. Though psoriasis and atopic dermatitis are usually benefited by exposure to sunlight, there are some instances in which this is not the case. Sunlight is a common precipitator of recurrences of herpes simplex, and in occasional persons this may be followed by a recurrence of erythema multiforme.

The distribution of lesions in photosensitivity reactions is always highly suggestive, but often not recognized promptly. It may be confused with a contact allergic reaction to an airborne contactant. Unilateral involvement may occasionally be noted, as, for instance, in involvement of the left forearm of a patient who is accustomed to riding in the left front seat of an automobile with an open window. In patients with photosensitivity reaction, the upper eyelids, postauricular and submental areas, scalp, palms and soles are spared. This is in contrast to reactions to an airborne contactant in which only the palms, soles, scalp and covered areas may be uninvolved.

The principal chemicals capable of producing phototoxic or photoallergic reactions when applied to the skin or ingested are as follows: psoralens; phenothiazines; salicylanilides and bithional, the use of which has been discontinued in soaps and creams in the United States; hexachlorophene, demeclocycline hydrochloride (Declomycin), all sulfanilamides, the antidiabetic sulfonylureas and the thiazides. Griseofulvin has been incriminated occasionally. In Table 14–2, the drugs and agents most commonly associated with photosensitivity reactions are summarized.

When confronted by a patient in whom there seems to be a possibility of a photosensitivity reaction, careful inquiry should be made in respect to all topical agents and ingested drugs. The likely responsible agent may become immediately apparent.

Although there is considerable discussion and some disagreement on the differentiation of phototoxic and photoallergic reactions, there can be no doubt that there are significant differences, and these are important in respect to the immediate and ultimate prognosis.

The varying types of sensitivity to light may be summarized as follows:

Normal (Sunburn). This is the type of reaction that any individual, other than dark-skinned blacks, will sustain in varying degrees on sufficient overexposure to midday sunlight. This may occur even if the sky is somewhat overcast. The burning effects of sunlight are much intensified by reflection from beach sand or snow. The activating wave lengths are between 290 and 320 nm.

Nonspecific (e.g., LE). In some patients with discoid LE, lesions

TABLE 14–1 SUNLIGHT-RELATED DISORDERS*

| Direct | | Indirect | | | | | | |
| Acute | Chronic | Exogenous Factor | | Endogenous Factor | | | | |
		Systemic Drugs	Topical Agents	Immunologic	Miscellaneous Primarily Cutaneous (Koebner's phenomena)	Biochemical Metabolic Nutritional Hormonal Enzymatic	Infectious (viral)	Genetic
Sunburn	Premature aging Premalignant lesions Malignant lesions	Photo-toxicity	Photo contact allergy; photo-toxicity	Lupus erythematosus Pemphigus erythematosus Solar urticaria Scleroderma Dermatomyositis (?)Polymorphic light eruption (?)Actinic reticuloid (?)Vitiligo	Psoriasis Lichen planus Keratosis follicularis Pityriasis rubra pilaris Erythema multiforme Rosacea	Solar urticaria Erythropoietic protoporphyria Porphyria cutanea tarda Porphyria(s) Pellagra Hartnup disease Phenylketonuria Hypopituitarism Hypogonadism Albinism	Herpes simplex Lymphogranuloma venereum Varicella	Xeroderma pigmentosum Bloom's syndrome Cockayne's syndrome Rothmund-Thomson syndrome Disseminated superficial porokeratosis Aminoacidurias

*Modified from Willis, I.: Sunlight and the skin. J.A.M.A. 217:1088–93, 1971.

tend to occur in areas most exposed to sunlight; in others it does not appear to be a factor. The mechanisms are obscure. In patients with systemic LE, the results of a sharp overexposure can be so disastrous as to make protection and avoidance very advisable. The patients should be protected from wave lengths between 290 and 320 nm.

True Photosensitivity. (See Table 14–3.) (a) Phototoxic. From idiopathic causes or as a result of applied or ingested drugs or other chemicals. (b) Photoallergic. Qualitative alteration. As in true contact allergic reactions, the combination of small amounts of the chemical and short exposure may elicit a sharp reaction.

Prevention

Photosensitivity reactions of all types tend to occur less during the winter months, particularly in temperate climates. In some of them, difficulty may be encountered only during the early part of the summer. In individuals with mild photosensitivity, common sense and the wearing of appropriate clothing is all that is necessary. The various sun-screen creams afford varying degrees of protection; these are available in a wide variety of proprietary preparations. Paraaminobenzoic acid and benzophene are the most widely used compounds. Zinc oxide or titanium oxide pastes are effective but cosmetically unacceptable.

In individuals with an extreme degree of photosensitivity, the wear-

TABLE 14–2 COMMON PHOTOSENSITIZING DRUGS AND AGENTS†

	Common Uses	Photosensitivity Reactions
Tetracyclines (mainly demeclocycline HCl)	Antibiotics	Ptx*
Sulfonamides	Antibacterials	Ptx; may induce PCA
Nalidixic acid	Antibacterial	Ptx
Griseofulvin	Antifungal	Ptx
Halogenated salicylanilides halogenated carbanilides halogenated phenols	Antibacterials in deodorant bar soap, antiseptics, cosmetics	PCA; mild Ptx
Phenothiazines	Sedatives, tranquilizers, antiemetics, antihistaminics, analgesic potentiators	Ptx; may induce PCA
Chlorothiazides	Diuretics	Ptx; may induce PCA
Sulfonylureas	Hypoglycemics	Ptx; may induce PCA
Furocoumarins	Melanogenics and in cosmetics	Ptx; may induce PCA
Coal tars, wood tars and petroleum products	Antipsoriatics and in cosmetics	Ptx; may induce PCA
Aminobenzoates	Sunscreens	PCA; ? mild Ptx

*Ptx signifies phototoxic reaction; PCA, photocontact allergic reaction.

†From Willis, I.: Photosensitivity. *In* Moschella, S. L., Pillsbury, D. M., and Hurley, H. J. (eds.): Dermatology, Vol. I. W. B. Saunders Co., Philadelphia, 1976, p. 332.

TABLE 14–3 CHARACTERISTICS OF PHOTOSENSITIVITY

Phototoxicity*		Photoallergy
Immediate	Delayed	
1) Usually associated with systemic medication, topically applied dyes, antibacterial agents and and tars or other endogenous factors.	1) Associated with topical and systemic use of furocoumarins.	1) Usually follows *repeated topical* exposure to photo-sensitizing chemicals.
2) Activating wavelengths and between 320 and 425 nm.	2) Activating wavelengths are between 320 and 400 nm.	2) Activating wavelengths are between 320 and 425 nm.
3) Requires *intense* light source.	3) Requires *intense* light source.	3) Requires *minute* quantities of light.
4) *Rapid* onset of burning, erythema and vesiculation. Occasionally bullae may form within 12 hours.	4) *Slow* onset of burning, erythema and vesiculation. First symptoms begin 6 to 12 hours *after* exposure and do not peak until 48 hours after exposure.	4) *Slow* onset of pruritus, erythema, edema oozing and crusting. Symptoms begin from 24 to 72 hours after exposure.
5) Resolution in 2 to 4 days with hyperpigmentation and desquamation.	5) Resolution is slow over a 7 to 14 day period with hyperpigmentation and desquamation.	5) Resolution is slow. One acute episode may resolve within 10 to 14 days. Persistent reactivity for many years is the rule.
6) Late sequelae or severe reactions may lead to scarring, hypopigmentation and lichenification.	6) Late sequelae consist primarily of hyperpigmentation.	6) Late sequelae include lichenification, acute flares, secondary infection and extreme discomfort that may last for years. Control may require complete avoidance of fluorescent lights and sunlight.
7) Histologically dermal edema, subepidermal bulla formation, perivascular lymphocytic infiltration and epidermal cell necrosis are seen acutely.	7) Histologically epidermal cell death, dyskeratosis and desquamation are most notable.	7) Histologically there is intraepidermal spongiosis and vesiculation and perivascular lymphocytosis. Eosinophils may be present.

*Rarely occurs in darkly pigmented individuals.

ing of appropriate protective clothing, however cumbersome and uncomfortable, is the only certain method. Some patients must remain indoors during daylight hours.

In polymorphic light eruptions and some other reactions, the administration of chloroquine in doses of 250 mg. daily may be useful, although its administration should be kept as short-term as possible because of the occasional toxic effects of this drug. An initial baseline ophthalmologic examination is essential, with checkups to detect retinopathy, which may at times be irreversible. Beta carotene (up to 180 mg. per day) is helpful in controlling the photosensitivity of erythropoietic protoporphyria. It is less effective in controlling other light-sensitive disorders, such as polymorphic light eruption, solar urticaria, porphyria cutanea tarda and hydroa aestivale.

PHOTOTHERAPY*

Since ancient times, physicians have empirically learned that sunlight exerts a beneficial effect on certain dermatoses. Even today, sunlight therapy, otherwise known as heliotherapy, is still a popular practice. Hundreds of patients are sent every year to certain geographic locales of high solar intensity, such as the Adriatic Coast or the Dead Sea area, for treatment and rehabilitation.

Sunlight would be the most convenient and economical light source were it not for the fact that it changes in intensity and quality, not only from season to season but also from day to day. Indeed, very often it is simply unobtainable. The development of artificial ultraviolet (UV) sources was therefore crucial in making phototherapy a realistic and available modality. The most elegant demonstration of the use of artificial UV radiation for the treatment of skin disease may be found in the early pioneering work of Niels R. Finsen. His success in controlling cutaneous tuberculosis, which at the time was a much dreaded disease, won him the Nobel Prize in Medicine in 1903.

The Solar Spectrum

Knowledge of the composition of solar energy reaching the earth's surface is important for understanding the responses of human skin to light. Units of measurement commonly in use are shown in Table 14–4. Two portions of the sun's electromagnetic spectrum are important in phototherapy: the ultraviolet (10 to 400 nm.) and the visible (400 to 720 nm.) regions. The former is conveniently divided into short UV (UV–C,

*By Kays H. Kaidbey, M. D., Assistant Professor of Dermatology, Hospital of the University of Pennsylvania, Philadelphia, Pa.

10 to 280 nm.), mid-UV (UV−B, 280 to 320 nm.) and long or near UV (UV−A, 320 to 400 nm.). Wavelengths below 290 nm. are efficiently absorbed by the ozone layer in the atmosphere and do not reach the surface of the earth. UV-B rays are responsible for the common sunburn reaction and can be blocked by ordinary window glass, which does not filter out the more penetrating UV-A. All UV wavelengths are capable of inducing erythema and pigmentation in human skin but differ strikingly in their biologic efficiency and in the quality of the responses they provoke. Thus, moderate doses of UV-B may produce blistering, whereas very large doses of UV-A usually elicit no visible changes. UV-C and UV-B erythema are characteristically delayed, peaking 8 and 24 hours after exposure respectively. UV-A and visible wavelengths are important because they are capable of initiating tissue damage by interacting with certain photoactive agents (photosensitizers), such as coal tar and psoralens. This principle is utilized to an advantage in phototherapy.

Artificial UV Sources

The most popular therapeutic UV radiation sources are basically mercury vapor arc lamps. A current is passed between electrodes separated by the mercury vapor, which is enclosed in a quartz or glass envelope. The discharge causes emission of radiation, the nature of which depends on the pressure of the mercury vapor. The radiation is further modified by "phosphors" applied to the inner surface of the glass envelope. Germicidal lamps (cold quartz) are low pressure mercury arcs, emitting primarily 254 nm. radiation. Medium pressure or hot quartz lamps (Hanovia Sunlamp, Kromayer) emit a line spectrum throughout the entire UV range. The fluorescent tubes are low pressure arcs in which the 254 lines

TABLE 14–4   THE MAJOR WAVELENGTH REGIONS OF THE SUN'S ELECTROMAGNETIC SPECTRUM

Region	Wavelength Range
Cosmic rays	5×10^{-5} nm.
Gamma rays	0.0005–0.14 nm.
X-rays	0.01–10 nm.
Short ultraviolet—UV-C	10–280 nm.
Mid-ultraviolet − UV-B	280–320 nm.
Long ultraviolet—UV-A	320–400 nm.
Visible	400–720 nm.
Near infrared	720 nm.–1.4 μ.
Middle infrared	1.5–5.6 μ.
Far infrared	5.6–1000 μ.
Microwaves and radio waves	1000 μ.–550 m.

10^{-6} meters $= 1$ Micron (μ.) $= 10^3$ Nanometers (nm.)
10^{-9} meters $= 1$ Nanometer (nm.) $= 1$) Angstroms (Å)

excite a special phosphor coating, causing it to fluoresce and radiate large amounts of UV at longer wavelenghts. These can be in the UV-B range, as in the common sunlamp tubes, or in the UV-A range, as in blacklight tubes, depending on the nature of the phosphor.

The amount of radiant energy impinging on the skin surface can be measured with a variety of radiometers and depends to a large extent on the power of the lamp and on the lamp-to-skin distance. The intensity of the radiation, or rate at which photons arrive at the skin surface, is commonly expressed in watts per square meter (W/m^2); whereas the dose of a given energy is expressed in Joules per square meter of skin surface (J/m^2). Biologic units are often employed in determining UV dosages. The minimal erythema dose (M.E.D.) is a popular and convenient, although highly variable determination, defined as the dose of radiation from a certain lamp required to elicit minimal (threshold) delayed erythema at a specified lamp-to-skin distance.

Phototherapy of Skin Diseases

A large number of cutaneous disorders have been treated with UV radiation and many claims of beneficial effects have been made. Only those in which phototherapy is of proven value will be discussed.

Psoriasis Vulgaris.   The beneficial effects of sunlight in psoriasis are primarily due to wavelengths in the UV-B range. Sunlight, however, is more effective than artificial UV-B sources. When the former is not available, total body exposures to UV-B radiation from fluorescent sunlamp tubes housed in specially designed cabinets can cause various degrees of regression of psoriatic plaques. Exposures should be administered daily, with a starting dose equal to the patient's M.E.D. Increments are adjusted so as to maintain minimal erythema of the normal skin. Overexposure may result in painful burns and flare-up of psoriasis (Koebnerization). Measures should always be taken to protect the eyes and sensitive skin areas prior to each exposure.

The therapeutic response to UV-B radiation is often slow and incomplete, so that other agents are almost always used concomitantly to enhance resolution. In the Goeckerman regimen, 1 to 6 per cent crude coal tar in petrolatum is applied to the entire body. The next day, excess tar is removed with gauze pads saturated with olive or cottonseed oil and the patient is exposed to UV radiation, either from a hot quartz mercury lamp or in a "sunlamp" cabinet. A soap and water bath is then given prior to fresh tar application. UV exposures are given daily and increments adjusted according to the patient's tolerance; enough dose is given to maintain minimal redness of the normal skin. Complications, such as tar folliculitis and flare-up of psoriasis (Koebnerization) from UV overdosage, are rarely encountered if treatment is expertly given. In the Ingram regimen, which is more popular in Europe, the patient is given a tar bath and then exposed to UV-radiation. The lesions are then covered with a zinc oxide paste containing 0.25 per cent to 1.0 per cent anthralin. Firm gauze dressings are used to keep the paste in position until the next UV exposure. Both of the above regimens are highly effective and result in satisfactory clearing in the majority of patients in about 3 weeks. They also require hospitalization, experienced personnel and trained nursing care. Other types of psoriasis, such as the pustular and exfoliative varieties, should not be treated with these regimens.

PHOTOCHEMOTHERAPY (PUVA).   This is a recently introduced, highly effective modality that entails the combined use of an orally administered photoactive drug, 8-methoxypsoralen followed by total body exposure to high intensity UV-A. 8-methoxypsoralen, a naturally occurring furocoumarin, is a potent photosensitizer activated by wavelengths around 360 nm. The excited molecule then combines covalently with thymine bases in DNA, thus presumably interfering with the rapidly replicating psoriatic cells. The drug is given at a dose of 0.4 to 0.7 mg. per kg. Two hours later, the patient is placed in a specially designed cabinet equipped with fluorescent tubes that emit UV-A. The starting dose is 1.0 to 2.0 Joules per cm.^{2}, increasing by 0.5 to 1.0 J per cm.^{2} depending on the patient's complexion and tolerance. Overdosage may result in serious blistering reactions and flare-up of psoriasis. Special goggles designed to filter out UV-A are worn on all treatment days. Exposures are limited to 2 or 3 times per week. About 80 per cent of patients will clear completely, but the number of treatments required varies from about a dozen to over 30. Remissions are shorter than those induced by the Goeckerman regimen, and maintenance exposures every week to 10 days are often necessary to keep the disease under control. PUVA is still an investigational procedure and the long-term side-effects are not fully determined. The advantage is that it is a clean treatment that does not require hospitalization.

Vitiligo.   Patients with vitiligo will occasionally respond favorably to treatment with oral psoralens followed by exposure to sunlight or artificial UV-A sources. The latter are to be preferred, since dosages are easy to monitor. The psoralens, usually 8-methoxypsoralen or trimethyl psoralen can be given orally or topically in an alcoholic solution. In the latter case, the concentration should not exceed 0.1 per cent. Topical therapy with sunlight is best avoided, since severe burns and blistering are almost unavoidable. Not more than 3 exposures per week should be given, since psoralen erythema, unlike sunburn, peaks in 48 to 72 hours. The initial UV-A dose should be individualized by determining the amount of energy required to elicit a minimal phototoxic reaction. As treatment progresses, adjustments are necessary, since the skin becomes more tolerant. Repigmentation is unpredictable and often incomplete, requiring prolonged therapy for over a year. The results are also influenced by the age of the patient and anatomical location of lesions, those over the face and trunk usually responding best.

Solar Urticaria.   Patients with solar urticaria can often be "desensitized" and made more tolerant to sunlight after repeated, carefully controlled exposures to artificial UV. The mechanism for this observed effect is unknown. Prior phototesting is essential in order to ascertain which wavelengths of the spectrum are responsible for provoking the symptoms (action spectrum). This will largely determine which UV-source should be employed for treatment. Daily total body exposures are given and dosages individualized. Once a state of tolerance is achieved, it can usually be maintained by regular daily exposures. Most patients experience good to excellent relief. The procedure has to be repeated yearly before each summer season.

Neonatal Hyperbilirubinemia.   Phototherapy of neonatal jaundice (from whatever cause) is currently a very popular modality and has significantly reduced the need for exchange transfusions. Its effectiveness is based on the fact that bilirubin is readily decomposed into several water soluble and excretable products by wavelengths in the visible range (400 to 500 nm.). Total serum levels of bilirubin, especially the unconjugated fraction, are effectively lowered. The yellow discoloration can often be seen to disappear in the exposed irradiated skin. Two light sources are commonly employed, a daylight fluorescent lamp and a special blue fluorescent lamp that has a higher output in the 400 to 500 nm. range. Exposure times vary from one center to another, and the most effective schedule has not been adequately worked out. The infant's eyes should always be protected.

Acne Vulgaris.   The majority of patients with acne vulgaris will experience some improvement after repeated exposure to sunlight. The effective wavelengths are in the UV-B range, although other wavebands may also be important. Artificial UV-B sources are less effective than natural sunlight. UV-erythema enhances resorption and resolution of pustules and inflammatory nodules but has no effect on comedones. A short course of phototherapy can be given using the fluorescent sunlamp tubes that are rich in UV-B. Irradiation is given daily and the dose gradually increased to maintain minimal erythema and desquamation. Phototherapy is usually given in conjunction with other antiacne measures. It should be kept in mind that sunlight occasionally aggravates acne in certain patients, for whom UV therapy should obviously be avoided.

REACTIONS TO COLD

The response of the skin to cold under varying conditions manifests itself in different ways. In frostbite, which may result from even brief exposures to extreme cold, the affected part becomes more or less anesthetized, with a whiteness that is characteristic. On rewarming there may be only erythema and some discomfort, but when marked tissue damage has occurred, blistering and ulceration may be seen. In severe cases, gangrene may result and amputation may become necessary.

The old method of treatment by rubbing snow on the affected area has now been discredited. It has now been established that rapid rewarming in a water bath at a temperature of from 104 to 107° F. is the best method. It should be continued for from 20 to 30 minutes. Subsequent treatment will depend upon the degree of tissue damage and vascular obstruction that has occurred.

Under certain conditions, prolonged exposure to cold temperatures above freezing may produce disabling changes. This is called trench foot because it occurs primarily in foot soldiers and was a widespread source of disability in Europe in World War II. The conditions that singly or in combination produce trench foot are cold temperatures (up to 10° F. above freezing), snug-fitting footgear, which allows little swelling of the feet, and continuously wet socks. In soldiers in combat, this combination may exist for days and nights on end. The affected foot feels cold and the sensation threshold is raised. On warming, there is vasodilatation and paresthesia. In some cases there may be superficial necrosis that looks alarmingly like true gangrene, but return to relative normality can be expected in time. The aftereffects are troublesome, including an inability to tolerate cold, increased sweating and evidence of vascular instability. Trench foot is almost completely preventable by the wearing of boots that allow some swelling of the feet without undue constriction and by regular changes to dry socks when they become wet. Heavy protective overshoes are also preventive.

Chilblains (Pernio)

Chilblains are rarely seen in the United States, where central heating is standard. During World War II, we saw many cases of chilblains in Britain, where central heating was not standard. It occurs during the cold months of early winter, principally in children and women.

The initial lesions consist of erythematous swelling, which may itch and which may lead to a mottled appearance of the skin. One cannot escape the feeling that chilblains and related disturbances are to some extent caused by alternate exposure to cold and to rather intense heat, as before a crackling hearth. Preventive measures include adequate protective clothing and an equable environmental temperature.

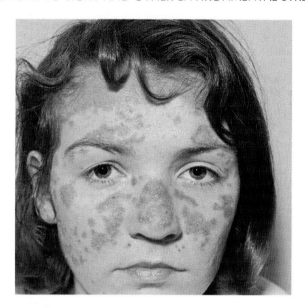

Figure 14–1.   Systemic lupus erythematosus

The affected skin areas were those receiving the largest amount of sunlight. The "butterfly" distribution on the nose and cheeks is classic.

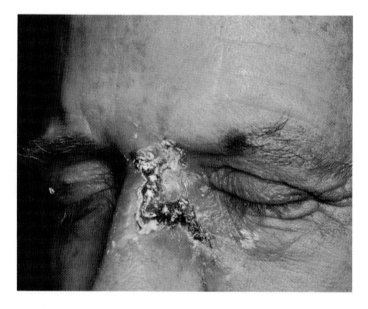

Figure 14–2.   Reaction in area of x-ray atrophy

This patient had received x-ray therapy for a basal cell epithelioma some years previously. He was exposed to sunlight sufficient to produce a moderate sunburn on normal skin, but a marked reaction developed in the area of x-ray atrophy.

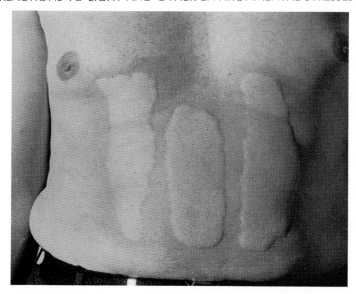

Figure 14–3. Cold urticaria

Marked urticarial lesion and erythematous flare in areas contacted with test tubes filled with ice water. Sudden body immersion in cold water would almost certainly produce severe histamine shock. The patient had chronic leukemia.

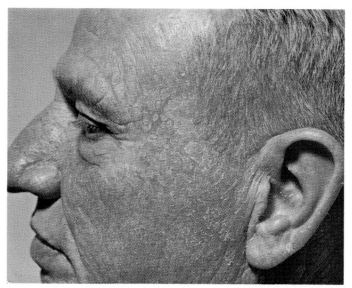

Figure 14–4. Photoallergic reaction

This patient was persistently reactive to very moderate exposure to sunlight. The exact cause was not determined.

15 | Drug Eruptions

With the introduction of a great many new compounds into medical practice during the past three decades, the variety and frequency of reactions to them appears to be increasing steadily, although in part this may be due to increased awareness by physicians of the possibility of such reactions and to more accurate tabulations in many hospitals. They constitute the largest single source of acute skin problems in hospitalized patients at the present time.

The skin is the organ most frequently affected, although other systems may be involved in reactions that are of great importance in terms of morbidity and mortality. These organs include the gastrointestinal tract, the liver, the kidney, the nervous system and the hematologic system. In any case of suspected drug reaction in the skin, the possibility of an even more important disturbance of some other organ system must be considered.

The wide variety of morphologic patterns of cutaneous drug reactions is seen in the following list.

From the rather bewildering number of drugs and the patterns of reactions to them, certain reactions may be selected as being most com-

TABLE 15-1   THE CLINICAL PATTERNS OF DRUG REACTIONS*

Fever	Lupus erythematosus syndrome
Urticaria	Acneiform eruptions
Serum sickness	Lichenoid eruptions
Anaphylactic shock	Pigmentation
Exanthematic eruptions	Ichthyosis
Scarlatiniform	Alopecia
Morbilliform	Change in hair colour
Exfoliative dermatitis	Agranulocytosis
Eczema	Aplastic anemia
Fixed eruptions	Haemolytic anemia
Bullous eruptions	Jaundice
Erythema multiforme	Nephrotoxicity
Purpura	Neurotoxicity
Phototoxic erythema	Carcinogenesis
Photoallergic eruptions	Teratogenic effects

*Rook, A., and Rowell, N. R.: Textbook of Dermatology, Vol. I. F. A. Davis Co., Philadelphia, 1968.

monly encountered in the case of each specific drug. It is to be emphasized, however, that in principle any drug may produce almost any type of cutaneous reaction.

Penicillin.   This compound and its synthetic analogues are responsible for many of the drug reactions currently encountered. The most frequent is urticaria, but bullous and eczematous responses may be seen. Penicillin is a strong sensitizer when applied to the skin and should *never* be used in this way. Penicillin is responsible yearly for many deaths from anaphylactic shock. In patients in whom penicillin sensitivity is suspected, administration by mouth is preferable, or, if parenteral administration is considered necessary, it should be given into the deltoid, where occlusion by tourniquet is feasible. In patients who have become sensitized to penicillin, recurrences of urticaria may result from ingestion of milk and milk products contaminated with tiny amounts of penicillin.

Chloramphenicol.   Skin reactions to this drug are infrequent and relatively minor. Its hematologic effects in the form of aplastic anemia, however, though uncommon, can be progressive and fatal. The administration of this drug must be restricted to infections that are grave and for which it is overwhelmingly the antibiotic of choice.

Aspirin.   In view of the extremely widespread use of this compound, the incidence of reaction to it must be very low. It must, however, always be considered as a possibility. It is such a part of the daily lives of some persons that they hardly think of it as a drug. Many food dyes and natural and artificial flavorings contain salicylates that may serve as direct histamine liberators or that may cross-react in patients who are allergic to aspirin to produce urticaria or anaphylaxis.

Sulfonamides.   Sulfonamide compounds *should not be applied topically*. If this is done, the individual may develop a severe dermatitis on later systemic administration. Sulfonamides are capable of producing fixed eruptions, erythema nodosum and, particularly in the case of long-acting compounds, very severe bullous eruptions involving the skin and mucous membranes, with a marked systemic reaction.

Griseofulvin.   This drug seldom produces clinically significant reactions in man if recommended doses are used. Transient macular erythemas may occur during the initial phase of therapy. Headaches, gastrointestinal upset, granulocytopenia, hepatocellular damage and photosensitivity have been seen during drug therapy, particularly if it is prolonged. It potentiates warfin-type anticoagulants and its absorption is depressed by barbiturates. Fortunately, absolute intolerance to the drug is rare.

Streptomycin.   Transitory rash may develop in some 5 per cent or more of patients, sometimes with fever, and rarely, exfoliative dermatitis. Urticaria and anaphylaxis are uncommon. Neurotoxicity, especially ototoxicity that is severe and permanent, may occur infrequently. Great care should be used when combining neurotoxic drugs. These reactions must be treated with respect, but it is often possible to resume the drug later without reaction. Vestibular damage is the most important untoward systemic reaction.

Tetracyclines.   Untoward reactions to these compounds are rare. Photosensitivity and light-induced onycholysis have been seen, particularly with demeclocycline hydrochloride (Declomycin). If possible, this group of drugs should be avoided in the pregnant female, infants and young children, since they may produce yellow staining and faulty enamel in the deciduous and developing permanent teeth.

Diphenylhydantoin (Dilantin).   A measles-like eruption is not infrequently noted during the first few weeks of treatment with this compound. Therapy may usually be resumed after the eruption has cleared. Psoriasiform eruptions, exfoliative dermatitis, bullous eruptions associated with phenytoin sodium or related compounds contraindicate reinstitution of therapy. Hyperglycemia, polyarthropathy, periarteritis nodosa, generalized lymphadenopathy and hirsuitism are infrequent complications, as are pancytopenia and toxic hepatitis. The most common and characteristic reaction is a gingival hyperplasia following prolonged administration. This may become so marked as to necessitate discontinuing the drug.

Oral Antidiabetic Agents (Sulfonylureas).   These compounds as a group are uncommon producers of skin reactions. More important, are occasional instances of granulocytopenia. Photosensitivity may be induced by some of them.

Antihistamines.   This group of compounds, which are very diverse in their chemical composition, is capable of causing a considerable variety of reactions. When used as topical anesthetics they frequently produce an allergic contact dermatitis. Skin reactions to systemically administered antihistamines are relatively uncommon. Of more importance are the side effects of drowsiness, headache and nausea. The patient should be warned about these possibilities on the initial administration. It is ordinarily possible, however, to select an antihistaminic compound that will be tolerated.

Synthetic Antimalarials.   Chloroquine, on being administered for malarial suppression, fortunately does not give rise to skin reactions very frequently. Long-term mepacrine (Atabrine) may produce a yellow discoloration of the skin that may be confused with jaundice. In mepacrine jaundice, however, the sclerae are spared. Pruritic pretibial hypertrophic lesions, clinically resembling lichen planus, are occasionally seen, but histologically the lesions have the morphology of a drug eruption. Preexisting psoriasis is frequently exacerbated by mepacrine.

Though corneal changes are seen following the administration of antimalarials, they are reversible and not serious. Of much more importance is a chorioretinitis, which may be noted after chloroquine has been administered for long periods, usually in daily doses greater than 250 mg.

Methotrexate.   This drug is occasionally used in severe psoriasis that is otherwise uncontrollable. It is a cytotoxic agent and therefore inherently dangerous. The most common reaction is one or more painful aphthous lesions of the mouth, which is an indication for immediate suspension of therapy. Cutaneous reactions on short-term administration are uncommon. Of much greater importance is bone marrow depression, and regular blood counts should be done. There is considerable risk of hepatic cirrhosis on long-term administration. Methotrexate is not a drug for casual or inexpert administration, and its justifiability in psoriasis is being severely questioned.

Inorganic Arsenical Compounds. Though long in disrepute, Fowler's solution is still occasionally administered in the treatment of psoriasis and dermatitis herpetiformis. Inhalation exposure may occur in some occupations, i.e., individuals using arsenic-containing sprays. The cutaneous lesions may require years to develop and consist of characteristic palmar or plantar keratoses and pigmentary changes on the trunk. The residual arsenic is a strong carcinogenic agent.

Barbiturates. The use of barbiturates is so widespread that instances of untoward reactions to them insofar as the skin is concerned must be very low. The possibility, however, should be considered. The eruption may be "fixed" to one or several small areas or be erythema multiforme–like in character and severity.

Phenothiazines. Phenothiazine compounds are represented by a wide variety of drugs, including psychotropic, antihistaminic and antipruritic agents. A fairly wide variety of skin reactions has been reported. Induced photosensitivity is the most striking of these. After prolonged administration in high doses, pigmentation of exposed areas of the skin may be noted, along with pigment in the eye.

Methoxsalen (8-MOP). This is a potent drug that is used in the treatment of idiopathic vitiligo, psoriasis and other light-responsive disorders. Its use is contraindicated in patients with liver disease or photosensitive disorders. Burns, often severe, of the skin, eyes and lips may result from limited exposures to sunlight or artificial UV-A light sources. The systemic use of methoxsalen should be limited to carefully controlled situations.

Gold Salts. Cutaneous reactions to injections of gold compounds are common and vary in their morphology.

Halogens. Iodides and bromides were used much more widely in medical therapy in years past, but they are still prescribed occasionally and may be found in some proprietary preparations. The most serious reaction to iodides is the anaphylactic type, occurring after the injection of radiographic contrast media.

Iodides are capable of producing a widespread acneiform eruption, bullous lesions, purpura or vegetating iododerma.

Bromoderma was seen very frequently in the past in the form of vegetating lesions resembling a tuberculous or blastomycetic granuloma. Development of these is ordinarily related to the taking of a fairly high dose over a prolonged period of time. Bromides are excreted slowly, and sodium chloride may be administered to hasten the process.

Teratogenic Effects of Drugs.   The thalidomide episode drew attention to the grave potentiality of administration of some drugs during the first trimester of pregnancy. The list of compounds capable of producing deforming effects on the fetus is by no means certain or complete. It is highly advised, however, that no drug that is not essential to the medical welfare of the mother be administered during pregnancy.

MANAGEMENT OF DRUG REACTIONS

In a patient sustaining a rash that might be attributable to a drug, the problem is a fairly simple one if only one drug is being taken, and this for a relatively short period of time. A high index of suspicion is advisable. It must be kept in mind that reactions may appear after a drug has been withdrawn for a week or two. Many patients, particularly those with chronic illnesses, especially psychiatric and cardiovascular, take a bewildering number of drugs. Precise data on the nature of each of these and the time at which each drug was started are often difficult to obtain, but an effort should be made to put these down as specifically as possible. Allergic reactions to drugs ordinarily occur within a week or two of the initial administration, but occasionally sensitization may not occur until the compound has been taken for weeks or many months.

There is no adequate and entirely certain method of testing for drug sensitivity, except in the case of topically applied compounds. Skin testing by scratch or intradermal methods yields a high proportion of false positive and false negative results, and in the case of penicillin sensitivity, may be hazardous.

In a patient suspected of having a drug reaction, elimination of all drugs is advisable, though this may be difficult or impossible in the case of lifesaving compounds. In any event, the number of drugs should be reduced to the absolute minimum.

Readministration of a drug that is suspected, but considered necessary to the welfare of the patient, should be very cautious and preferably it should be given by mouth, with an initial dose that is very small in relation to the usual one.

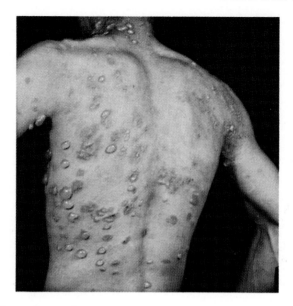

Figure 15–1.   Bullous sulfonamide reaction

Severe pemphigus-like drug eruption, with high fever, and oral-pharyngeal lesions induced by a single tablet of sulfathiazole. The patient had been sensitized originally by application of a sulfa cream for chronic folliculitis of the beard.

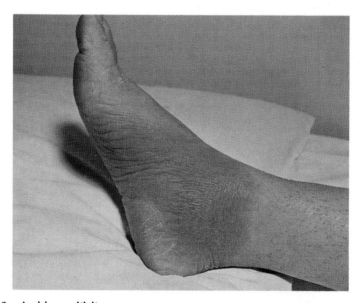

Figure 15–2.   Aspirin sensitivity

In listing the drugs they are taking many patients do not include aspirin. Moreover, W. B. Shelley has listed some 51 combinations of drugs or flavorings that contain salicylates, along with numerous sun-tan lotions and common home plants.

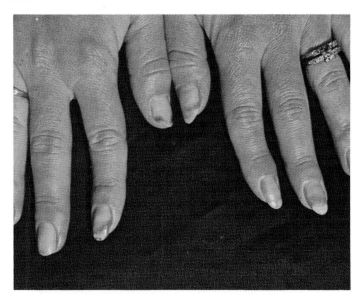

Figure 15–3. Tetracycline reaction – nails

Yellowing and some separation of the distal portion of the fingernails in patient taking a tetracycline. Some phototoxic reaction appeared to be involved.

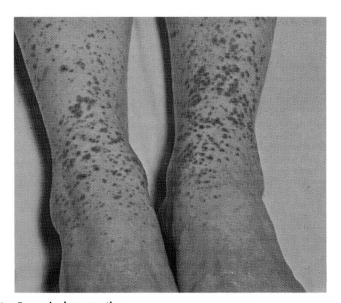

Figure 15–4. Purpuric drug reaction

This reaction occurred in a patient on iodide therapy. There were no hematologic changes.

16

Bacterial Infections

THE NORMAL BACTERIAL FLORA OF THE SKIN

The skin has a large population of bacteria — so many, in fact, that one cannot escape the notion that these usually harmless organisms play some beneficent role in the physiology of the skin. The normal skin bacteria are concentrated in hair follicles and in moist intertriginous areas. These are principally *Staphylococcus epidermidis*. In areas of skin with a high concentration of sebaceous glands, anaerobic *Corynebacteria* may be recovered in abundance. Fungi of the genus *Candida* may sometimes be recovered from nondiseased skin. The bacterial population of the skin is far from homogeneous; in intertriginous areas, for instance, aerobic diphtheroids may be predominant. The toe webs, particularly under tropical conditions, have a remarkably varied microflora, including such gram-negative organisms as species of *Pseudomonas, Klebsiella* and *Proteus;* gram-positive bacilli, such as species of *Corynebacteria;* and species of *Candida*.

Streptococci are almost never isolable from normal skin. Coagulase-positive staphylococci are occasionally encountered, but usually only in small numbers. In skin inflamed in various ways, particularly chronic dermatitis, the change in the bacterial flora is striking. Coagulase-positive staphylococci may now be recovered frequently and in abundance, although they may not be producing overt disease.

The prevention of bacterial infection is largely dependent on two overriding factors — *dryness* and *good hygiene*. Skin that is constantly moistened by sweat, occlusion and immersion becomes extremely vulnerable to invasion by pathogenic micro-organisms. Drying is the principal mechanism by which the skin prevents overpopulation by bacteria. Simple occlusion of the skin by an impermeable material such as polyethylene film (Saran Wrap) results in a very rapid increase in its bacterial population.

Soap and water bathing is the most effective means of "degerming" the skin. This is accomplished by detergent action, not antibacterial. The advantages of soaps containing a bactericidal agent in preventing infections of the skin are uncertain, although the so-called germicidal soaps may incorporate antibacterial chemicals as an attractive gimmick. In the past many of these soaps contained halogenated salicylanilides, which have been shown to be associated with both contact allergy and photosensitivity.

The management of mild abrasions, scratches and superficial cuts of the skin has possibly been the object of more unscientific attention than any other aspect of minor medicine. *The most important first-aid measure is thorough cleansing with soap and water.* Dirt or other debris should be meticulously rinsed away. The application of tincture of iodine or organic mercurial solutions has long been outmoded; there was never any convincing proof of their efficacy. Nor is there solid evidence that the prophylactic application of antibiotic creams is of value. Some persons may have contact allergies to them, and greasy ointments may impede the development of a protective adherent crust.

If the superficial injury is at a site subject to further mechanical injury, a protective dressing may be necessary. This should not be occlusive and should be changed often enough to prevent its becoming soggy.

Puncture wounds or significant lacerations requiring surgical management are, of course, in a different category, but the principles of thorough initial cleansing and avoidance of too occlusive dressings still hold. In any significant puncture wound, a booster injection of tetanus toxoid is advisable.

INFECTIONS

Bacterial infections constitute a significant and extremely important segment of dermatology. Both macro and micro enviromental conditions play a major role in determining the anatomical location, severity and duration of infections. Warm, moist climates; occlusive clothing and footwear; moist, closely opposed skin surfaces; and constant exposure to water predispose to a profound overgrowth of bacteria and subsequent infection. These factors are all amplified in diabetic and immunologically compromised patients. Elaborate modification of the environment and careful skin hygiene may be necessary if repeated infections are to be avoided.

The principal types of cutaneous bacterial infections are:

Impetigo.   The suffix "contagiosa" is commonly applied to this infection. It is highly contagious among the newborn in nurseries and in young children but becomes less so in older persons. Impetigo is characterized by an initial short-lived vesicopustule or bulla that is succeeded by a superficial crust. This may be followed, especially in areas of trauma, by deeper erosion or ulceration (ecthyma).

If cultured early in its course, impetigo *ordinarily* yields Group A beta-hemolytic streptococci. These are promptly joined by staphylococci. The initial organism is the chief cause for concern, because it is a virulent source of glomerulonephritis.

TREATMENT.   The superficial nature of early impetigo invites dependence on topical antibiotic therapy. In impetigo of any significant extent, however, particularly in children, concomitant systemic antibiotic therapy should be administered, preferably penicillin V for oral treatment, parenteral crystalline penicillin G for initial treatment of severe infections, parenteral procaine penicillin G for less severe infections and parenteral benzathine penicillin G for the prophylaxis of rheumatic fever or Group A streptococcal pharyngitis. Erythromycin or the cautious use of a cephalosporin may be required in individuals who are allergic to penicillins.

Bacterial infection may occur secondary to some other skin disturbance. Contact dermatitis, acute dermatophytosis, bullous eruptions of all types, seborrheic dermatitis, nummular dermatitis, burns and intertrigo are particularly prone to bacterial infection. This may occur in an easily recognizable form such as impetigo or cellulitis, but frequently it develops insidiously. The bacterial population of a chronically inflamed area of skin is frequently very different from that of normal skin. It may become very mixed, with organisms such as *Proteus*, *Herellea* and *Pseudomonas* entering the picture.

Ecthyma.   Ecthyma is essentially ulcerated impetigo. The depth of the ulcer varies. It is usually covered by a crust that is more or less adherent. There are varying degrees of cellulitis surrounding the ulcer. New lesions may develop at sites of mild trauma.

The bacterial population of ecthyma is often mixed — coagulase-positive staphylococci and Group A beta-hemolytic streptococci. In humid tropical environments, ecthyma must be regarded with great respect; such lesions may become quite destructive. In a single low-grade lesion without significant surrounding cellulitis, it may be justifiable to depend on the application of an antibacterial cream 3 times daily. If there is significant inflammation, systemic antibiotic therapy is indicated.

Folliculitis, Furuncles and Carbuncles.   Staphylococcal infections of this type have their origin in the hair follicles. In folliculitis, the inflammation is superficial, although many follicles may be involved. Follicular irritation, as in ingrown hairs, may occur in the absence of any significant bacterial invasion.

A furuncle is characterized by acute inflammation arising deep in one or more hair follicles. The onset is announced by tenderness, pain and surrounding cellulitis. Within a few days the boil "points" and drains, often spontaneously and without need for surgical drainage. This may be the end of the infection, but frequently "satellite" lesions develop in the region of the original furuncle or elsewhere.

TREATMENT.   The time-honored local treatment of a boil is hot wet compresses. This may accelerate "pointing" and reduce discomfort.

Prompt systemic antibiotic therapy is ordinarily indicated, initially with a penicillinase-resistant penicillin, erythromycin or cephalosporin. When material for culture becomes available, the identity of the organism and its antibiotic sensitivities should be determined, particularly in hospital-acquired infections in which the incidence of antibiotic-resistant staphylococcal infections may be high.

For reasons not readily apparent, some otherwise healthy young adults are subject to repeated bouts of disabling boils. In such individuals, a careful search should be made for underlying predisposing diseases, such as diabetes, lymphomas or other factors leading to immune compromise. Staphylococcal vaccines and toxoids are of no demonstrated value in preventing new lesions. The use of antibacterial soaps or surgical scrub mixtures may possibly be of some value in preventing new lesions. Heavy irritating gear, which may be sweaty and bacteria ridden, or sweat shirts may be factors in perpetuating the infections.

A *carbuncle* is a deep infection of a number of adjacent hair follicles. A common site is on the posterior neck. This lesion, even with well-selected antibiotic and surgical therapy, may be very destructive, especially in older, debilitated patients. It can be fatal.

Erythrasma. This scaling, circinate, mildly inflamed eruption is easily confused with a fungal infection. It is encountered most commonly in subtropical and tropical climates. The causative organism is *Corynebacterium minutissimum*, a bacterium that is sensitive to broad spectrum antibiotics. The infection is demonstrable by a coral-red fluorescence when examined under a Wood's light.

Hidradenitis Suppurativa. This is an uncommon but often very chronic infection of the apocrine glands, which are found principally in the axillae and anogenital region. The lesions appear as recurrent deep furuncle-like lesions that are painful and disabling. If the infection is recognized early and vigorous antibiotic therapy and appropriate surgical drainage carried out, the infection may be checked. In some instances, however, relapses may be encountered for months or years, and excision and grafting of the affected areas may become necessary in order to remove the resultant sinus tracts.

Swimming Pool Granulomas. *Mycobacterium balnei (M. marinum)* is a photochromogen that may contaminate some fish tanks, swimming pools and larger bodies of water such as the Chesapeake Bay. Traumatic inoculation of the organism results in a chronic granuloma that is very similar clinically and histologically to tuberculosis. Therapy may include surgical debridement as well as chemotherapy with rifampin and ethambutol hydrochloride. The old first-line antituberculous drugs tend to be ineffective.

Intertrigo. Intertrigo is defined as an eruption of the skin produced by friction and occlusion of adjacent surfaces. Characteristically, the axillae, inframammary folds, groin, toe webs and redundant skin folds are involved. Heat, moisture, sweat retention and friction combine to create an ideal environment for micro-organic growth. Bacteria, yeast and fungi may synergistically produce loss of epithelium and ulceration. Group A beta-hemolytic streptococci may invade the ulcerations. *Pseudomonas* species and *Candida albicans* produce unusually destructive lesions in the toe webs. Therapy consists of cleaning frequently, minimizing skin surface friction and occlusion, creating a cool as well as a dry environment with cotton or wool pledgets and specifically treating the identified pathogenic micro-organisms. Secondary underlying disorders, such as contact dermatitis, must also be identified and treated specifically.

Erysipeloid.   This is an infection caused by *Erysipelothrix rhusiopathiae* that occurs principally in fishermen and fish dealers, meat dressers and kitchen workers. The most common form is the development of erythema and edema at a site of injury, such as from a fishhook. The inflammation spreads peripherally, and vesicles or a bulla may develop. Systemic symptoms are ordinarily lacking, but generalized forms may occur, with a generalized rash, joint pains and endocarditis. Penicillin and other antibiotics are usually effective.

Erysipelas.   This is a characteristic type of superficial cellulitis in which an edematous, brawny, infiltrated circumscribed plaque develops and spreads peripherally. It was fairly common in pre-sulfonamide days but has now become quite rare, probably because the initial lesion from which it develops is recognized promptly and is treated by effective antibacterial measures. It is a disease of great historical significance because of its recognition as a source of fatal puerperal fever and its role in the beginnings of the enormously significant "bacterial age" of medicine. Vesicles and bullae may develop, and systemic symptoms of fever and toxicity are common. The causative bacterium is beta-hemolytic streptococcus. Penicillin therapy is promptly curative.

Recurrent Cellulitis (Elephantiasis Nostras).   Elephantiasis nostras is a highly characteristic type of recurrent cellulitis, usually of the lower leg, in which repeated inflammatory episodes lead to lymphatic obstruction and increasing permanent edema. The syndrome is often extraordinarily resistant to treatment, which consists of vigorous antibiotic therapy with the onset of each episode of cellulitis, bed rest and supportive bandaging. Careful assessment of lymphatic and venous circulation should be carried out, along with repeated examination for any lesion of the foot, particularly between the toes, that might serve as a portal of entry. Continued compressive support between attacks is advisable.

Leprosy.   "Leprosy is a chronic infectious disease of man, caused by *Mycobacterium leprae*, affecting chiefly the skin, mucous membranes and certain peripheral nerves. Man is the only known source of infection. Two major types are recognized, lepromatous and tuberculoid, and in addition to these, an indeterminate or uncharacteristic form. Tuberculoid lesions occasionally become lepromatous, passing through a 'borderline' stage. Indeterminate lesions may progress to become either tuberculoid or lepromatous. Death is usually due to other causes. In the lepromatous type, life is shortened by various complications, of which tuberculosis and secondary amyloidosis are prominent. In the tuberculoid type, life expectancy is unaffected."*

---

*Doull, J. A.: Veterans Admin. Tech. Bull. 10:98, Washington, D.C., March 1954. An exceedingly informative summary of modern leprology.

Leprosy is possibly the world's most common chronic infection. As of 1970, it is estimated that there are not less than 10 million cases throughout the world.* But physicians in temperate areas will almost never encounter a case; in the U.S.A. in 1968, only 147 new infections were reported. The areas of highest incidence include parts of China, Japan, Korea, Iran, Turkey, Greece, Portugal, Romania, Spain, USSR, Algeria, Egypt, Morocco, Libya and the Union of South Africa.

The signs and symptomatology of leprosy are so diverse as to make summarization difficult. A brief listing is as follows.

LEPROMATOUS TYPE.   Infectious Hansen's bacilli are demonstrable in lesions. Nasal obstruction and epistaxis are common early signs. The initial lesions may be erythema nodosum. The first skin lesions are macular, with an ill-defined border. Localized and diffuse infiltration of the skin and mucous membranes develops slowly, in papules, nodules and plaques. Eye lesions are common. Destruction of the nasal septum may occur.

TUBERCULOID TYPE.   Lepra bacilli are not found in lesions, except during acute exacerbations, and then with difficulty. The lepromin test is positive, showing an immune response. The initial skin lesions are macular, sometimes showing only hypopigmentation. The margins are sharp. Impairment of sensation occurs early. Polyneuritis occurs in all types of leprosy, most commonly in the tuberculoid. This is evidenced by tingling and numbness, weakness and atrophy of muscles, particularly those of the hand. Decalcification of bones may occur. A perforating ulcer of the foot is a troublesome complication.

THE INDETERMINATE TYPE.   In this type of leprosy there is no clearcut differentiation on the basis of signs, the lepromin test, recovery of bacilli and the pathologic picture, and time must elapse before the classification becomes more precise.

Biologic false positive tests for syphilis occur in leprosy and may lead to diagnostic error.

The treatment of leprosy with the use of Dapsone (DDS), corticosteroids, B-663 (Geigy) and cyclophosphamide has improved, but the response is usually discouragingly slow. It is best directed by a physician with broad experience in dealing with the disease.

---

*Personal communications, Dr. Esmond R. Long.

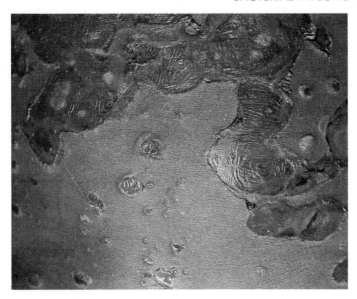

Figure 16–1.   Bullous impetigo

Extensive bullae formation, with numerous rapidly developing satellite lesions. Systemic antibiotic injection essential—preferably a penicillin or erythromycin. A single injection of benzathine penicillin G is often curative.

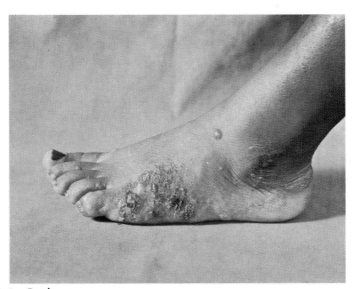

Figure 16–2.   Pyoderma

Mixed secondary infection of area of dermatitis on foot. Note new vesicular lesions that are developing. Bed rest advisable. The patient should avoid occlusive footwear.

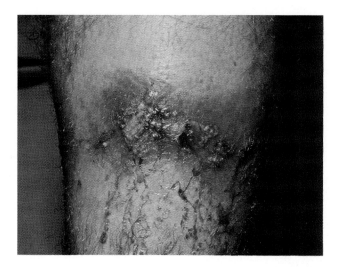

Figure 16–3.   Mixed infection with Staphylococcus aureus and B. hemolytic streptococci

Combined cellulitis and ecthyma. The vivid peripheral erythema is highly suggestive of streptococcal infection. The bacteria-laden drippings are obviously highly infectious.

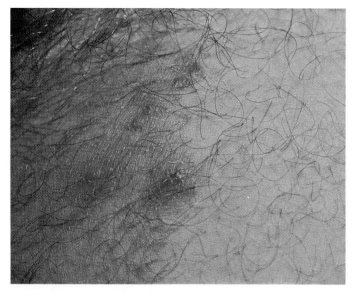

Figure 16–4.   Furuncles

The furuncles are invading an area of low-grade tinea cruris. Any area of skin inflammation particularly in hairy areas, is susceptible to furunculosis. Once established, the infection may tenaciously resist dislodgment.

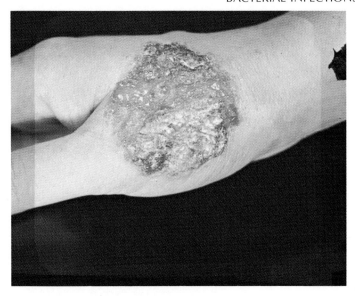

Figure 16–5.   Secondarily infected nummular dermatitis

The presence of bacterial infection here is clearly evident. In many cases of secondary infection, however, it is much more subtle. *Staphylococcus aureus* is the most frequently found pathogen.

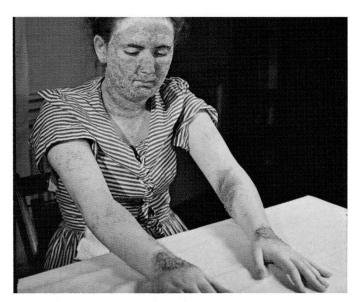

Figure 16–6.   Secondary infection — atopic dermatitis

Low-grade inflammation and secondary infection in chronic eczema. The principal primary focus of infection is commonly in fissures about the ears and neck. Patients with extensive disease are frequently colonized with large numbers of *Staphylococcus aureus* In excess of 75 per cent of these people are nasal carriers.

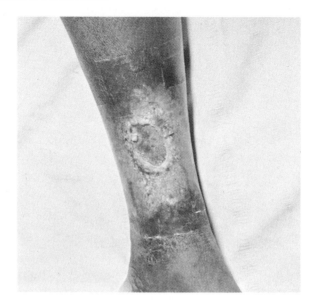

Figure 16–7.   Ulcer in patient with peripheral vascular disease

While the underlying vascular changes are principally responsible, bacterial infection may play an important secondary role. In longstanding ulcers, malignant changes may be suspected.

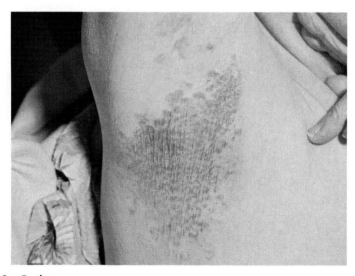

Figure 16–8.   Erythrasma

Only in recent years has this fungal-like infection been established as bacterial — *Corynebacterium minutissimum*. Responsive to oral antibiotic therapy.

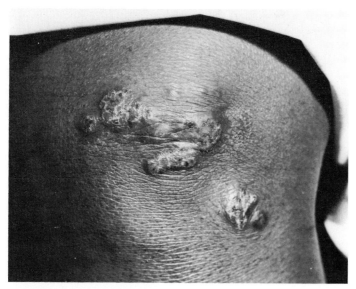

Figure 16–9.   Swimming pool granulomas

This infectious granuloma followed traumatic inoculation of *Mycobacterium balnei (marinum)* from water of a contaminated recreational pool finished in native stone. Fish tanks may also be a source of the infection.

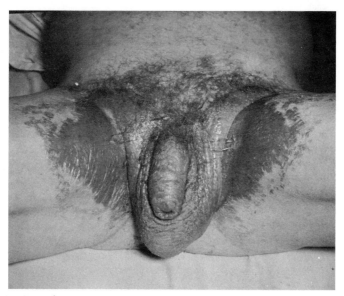

Figure 16–10.   Intertrigo

This diabetic patient has an acute mixed infection of the groin. Note that the lesions occur on opposing skin surfaces, thus illustrating the importance of rubbing in lesion development. *Candida* species and *Pseudomonas* species were in the mixed isolates taken from the affected areas.

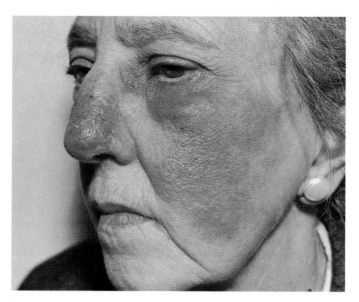

Figure 16–11.   Erysipelas

A relatively superficial streptococcal cellulitis. Penicillin therapy ordinarily produces a rapid cure. Formerly quite common, this infection has become rare in general practice.

17

Fungal and Yeast Infections

Superficial infections of the skin by fungi (principally *Trichophyton mentagrophytes* and *Trichophyton rubrum*) and by yeasts (*Monilia, Candida*) constitute a large section of clinical dermatology. Fungi, which are microscopic plants, tend to remain in the horny surface of the skin, although there are organisms that are primarily systemic. The fungi of chief dermatologic significance are members of the genera *Trichophyton, Microsporum* and *Epidermophyton*.

DISEASES DUE TO FUNGI

The inflammation caused by superficial fungi varies from slight scaling and occasional fissuring between the toes, to more extensive dry reddish scaling, to acute vesicular and bullous flare-ups — most commonly on the feet — and occasionally to angry red granulomas, particularly if the fungi have been implanted from an animal source.

Ringworm Infections of the Glabrous Skin

The only ringworm infection in which a diagnosis can be made almost entirely on clinical grounds is that caused by *T. rubrum*. In this very chronic infection, the hand or sole, as a rule, shows a dull red, low-grade inflammation with moderate dry scaling. On the foot the distribution is much like a low-cut moccasin. The infection may remain localized to one foot or one hand for years. Other parts of the body often remain uninvolved, except in the case of environmental conditions of heat and high humidity or in patients with debilitating systemic diseases, such as uncontrolled diabetes, Cushing's syndrome, or lymphoma, in whom the infection may become very extensive.

Another type of fungal infection, usually caused by *T. mentagrophytes*, is suggestive clinically, but the diagnosis cannot be made with certainty in the absence of microscopic demonstration of the fungi. This is the type in which there is recurrent itching and scaling between the toes,

243

most frequently in the fourth interspace, and vesicles and scaling on the soles. The infection is subject to acute flare-ups, particularly during warm weather and when occlusive footgear is worn.

All types of fungal infections have a tendency to much wider dissemination under conditions of poor hygiene, heat and humidity. This frequently presents as inflamed annular and circinate lesions of various portions of the body, particularly the buttocks, inner thighs and lower trunk. At times the inflammation may become very diffuse, simply myriads of tiny punctate inflamed papules without the formation of ring-shaped lesions.

KOH Examination. Laboratory confirmation of a diagnosis of a ringworm infection is easily achieved by the following procedure.

1. The affected area is scraped with a dull scalpel, or the top of a blister is cut away with curved scissors. It is convenient to scrape scales onto a folded piece of black paper.

2. The scales or bulla top are placed on a slide, and 10 per cent to 20 per cent KOH solution dropped onto the material.

3. The slide is gently warmed over an open flame.

4. The slide is examined microscopically. If the scales are relatively thin, mycelia are promptly visible if present. In thicker scales, or in pieces of nail plate, more time may be necessary for adequate keratolysis.

(Caution: Potassium hydroxide solution is hard on microscopes. Expensive new scopes should not be used for KOH examinations.)

Ringworm Infection of Nails

In any long-standing ringworm infection of the hands or feet, involvement of the nails occurs almost inevitably. It may occur without prior visible involvement of the skin. The nails become distorted and thickened, with an increase in scaling under the nail plate. Such infection is occasionally difficult to differentiate from the nail changes seen in psoriasis and, less frequently, lichen planus and alopecia areata. Prior to the availability of griseofulvin, ringworm infection of the nails was almost impossible to cure, and a cure is still achieved with difficulty, even after months of griseofulvin therapy.

Ringworm Infections of the Scalp (Tinea Capitis)

This type of infection, which is almost entirely confined to children, was formerly seen in epidemic proportions in many population centers, most frequently among the underprivileged and among residents of orphanages and other institutions. Probably as a result of relatively simple cure by griseofulvin, even when given in a single large dose, tinea capitis is now much less common.

Differential Diagnosis of Ringworm Infection

Superficial ringworm infections of the skin must be differentiated from several other inflammatory conditions of the skin. These are:

Yeast Infections. (Discussed below.)

Intertrigo. An inflammatory condition produced by maceration of the skin in body folds, particularly in obese individuals. Mechanical factors often play a greater role in this condition than infectious agents.

Erythrasma. (See Chapter 16, Bacterial Infections.)

Because of the capacity of fungi to localize and produce inflammation of the skin in various restricted areas, the terms Tinea cruris, and Tinea corporis have come into common use. The course of these infections is entirely comparable, varied by special physiologic conditions in the particular part involved.

Tinea Versicolor. This is a very common condition affecting the trunk and upper portions of the extremities in varying degree. The causative organism is probably not a yeast but rather a fungus. The lesions consist of lightly scaling, round patches about 1 cm. in diameter. The color varies from fawn to brown. The affected areas become most apparent if the patient becomes tanned. The lesions themselves fail to pigment and remain as whitish macules that may be in rather marked contrast to the surrounding pigmented skin.

Tinea versicolor is symptomless, and treatment is ordinarily not required. If, however, the patient is insistent that something be done, washing the affected areas with selenium sulfide shampoo twice a week is ordinarily effective, though eventual recurrence is the rule. Clotrimazole (Lotrimin) 1 per cent cream or solution applied twice daily usually produces effective results within 2 to 4 weeks.

Wood's Light Examination. This special equipment for the detection of several types of superficial infection is available in most large medical installations. Ultraviolet light is filtered through Wood's glass, which is composed of barium silicate containing 9 per cent nickel oxide.

Tinea capitis caused by certain fungi, particularly *Microsporum audouini*, shows a brilliant greenish fluorescence. This is of inestimable value in surveying groups of individuals in which the infection may have become endemic. However, no fluorescence is seen in *Trichophyton tonsurans* infections.

Tinea versicolor also fluoresces under the Wood's light, and the extent of the infection may prove to be much greater than evident on inspection in ordinary light.

Erythrasma fluoresces a coral red, which is of great usefulness in detecting this superficial bacterial infection.

Treatment

Until the advent of griseofulvin, the treatment of superficial fungal infections was unsatisfactory. This situation is now much changed, although in fungal infections of the nails, particularly the toe nails, very long courses of this antibiotic are necessary, and complete cure without recurrence is almost impossible to achieve.

It is very advisable that a diagnosis of fungal infection be confirmed by demonstration of the organism before treatment with griseofulvin is started. There may be instances, however, in which the clinical signs are so suggestive and laboratory facilities so lacking that a "therapeutic trial" may be justifiable.

Griseofulvin should be administered only in the micronized form, because it is absorbed better from the gastrointestinal tract. The absorption is further increased if the drug is given after a meal, particularly one containing a fair amount of fat. The dose is 1 to 2 gm. daily, the latter ordinarily being the preferred initial dose. In very acute flare-ups of dermatophytosis, in which there is a large element of sensitivity to the fungus, griseofulvin may not be rapidly effective, and a short supplementary course of corticosteroid may be indicated. It is important that if griseofulvin proves effective, it not be discontinued too soon, i.e., after only a week of treatment. In proven fungal infections, administration over a period of at least 4 weeks is advisable to control a tendency to recurrence.

Like any drug, griseofulvin may produce unwanted reactions. The principal reactions are skin rashes, urticaria, gastrointestinal disturbances and headache. However, patients receiving prolonged treatment should have periodic monitoring of renal, hepatic and hemopoietic systems. Phototoxic reactions and cross reactivity with penicillin have been described. Granulocytopenia is among the most severe side effects. Should any of these untoward symptoms be noted, suspension of the drug, at least temporarily, is advisable. It is frequently possible to resume griseofulvin therapy without subsequent recurrence of the reaction.

After the infection is under control it is important to carry out measures designed to prevent relapse. Hygiene should be as scrupulous as possible, including daily bathing if possible and thorough drying of the skin, particularly of the intertriginous surfaces. In infections of the feet, open sandals should be worn if conditions permit.

Although dusting powders and creams containing fatty acids have been widely used in the prevention of fungal infection, their advantages over a simple nonmedicated powder are uncertain. Tolnaftate (Tinactin) cream or lotion is useful and may assist in preventing recurrences. More recently, clotrimazole (Lotrimin) and similar topical preparations have been of value in initiating cures and preventing recurrences. Under conditions that are favorable to recurrence of fungal infections, U.S. Army experience in Vietnam would indicate that the prophylactic administration of griseofulvin, 0.5 to 1.0 gm. daily, 5 times weekly has considerable value.

Among older preparations that still have some usefulness are the following:

1. Dilute Whitfield's ointment
Salicylic acid	2 to 3 per cent (not more)
Benzoic acid	4 per cent
Hydrophilic ointment	q.s.

2. Thymol
Thymol	1 per cent
Salicylic acid	3 per cent
Propylene glycol	q.s.

3. Carbol fuchsin paint (Castellani)
   (Especially for intertriginous areas)
   Follow with dusting powder when paint dries.

Many others could be cited. It is extremely important that such preparations not have irritant or sensitizing properties.

Under poor hygienic conditions and a warm environment, extensive superficial fungal infections may not be controlled until the patient is removed to better facilities and surroundings.

CANDIDIASIS (MONILIASIS)

Yeast-like fungi are commonly found on the skin, particularly chronically inflamed skin. They are regularly a part of the gastrointestinal flora. There is frequently an increase of *Candida* in the mouth and vagina after broad spectrum antibiotic therapy. Although yeasts such as *Candida albicans* are undoubtedly capable of producing inflammation under certain circumstances and may produce systemic infections in debilitated patients, demonstration of the organism on diseased skin does not necessarily mean that it is a primary etiologic factor.

Candidae tend to flourish in moist warm areas of the body. They also tend to grow profusely in areas that are otherwise diseased, particularly in patients with congenital ectodermal defects. In the following clinical conditions, *Candida* is seen playing a predominant role, if not the sole one:

Thrush, candidiasis of the mouth in infants, was much more common in the past than is now the case. It occurs as curd-like, friable, well-defined areas in the mouth. Removal of the whitish substance reveals an underlying red inflammation.

Candida may be recovered in intertrigo, seborrheic dermatitis and psoriasis in intertriginous areas. Flare-ups may occur in the form of increased redness and fissuring in the fold, with superficial satellite pustules. This is most often seen in warm humid environments and particularly in obese patients.

Candida may affect the paronychial margins of the fingernails, resulting in a rather marked deformity of the nail plate. This is most likely to occur in persons whose hands are in water a great deal, such as cooks, maids, bartenders and housewives.

Candidiasis may also be seen in a generalized distribution, usually with accompanying inflammation of the lips and mouth. In such cases some underlying factor is almost always present, either a congenital abnormality of the skin or a significant systemic disease.

Treatment

For the topical treatment of candidiasis, nystatin is possibly the sovereign remedy in lotion, cream or ointment form. Amphotericin B is also effective. It is sometimes used with a corticosteroid preparation, and this may increase its anti-inflammatory effects. Clotrimazole (Lotrimin) and similar compounds are available as creams, ointments and vaginal tablets and are effective in the topical management of yeast infections. Under no circumstances should occlusive dressings be used in yeast-infected areas, because this favors the growth of the yeast and the release of the irritating endotoxin that it produces.

Among the older remedies for candidiasis is gentian violet, best applied in an aqueous solution of 0.5 to 1 per cent. It is messy in the extreme.

THE DEEP MYCOSES

Certain fungal infections have the capacity to invade systemically after being inoculated into the skin or after being inhaled. These are called the *deep* fungal infections in contrast to the *superficial* dermatophytic infections, which remain in the superficial portions of the skin. Deep fungal infections are rarely seen by the general physician, except in certain regions. Sporotrichosis is almost epidemic among gold miners in South Africa, where the mine beams support an abundant growth of the fungus. In much lesser incidence, it has a worldwide distribution. Coccidioidomycosis is endemic in certain dry sandy areas of the southwest United States, and a high proportion of the residents develop signs of the primary infection, although they may not be recognized as such. Blastomycosis is seen principally in the central United States. South American blastomycosis, as the name indicates, is encountered in Central and South America and in Cuba.

The principal features of these deep fungal infections may be summarized as follows.

Blastomycosis

The most common portal of infection is the skin. The entrance of the organism (*Blastomyces dermatitidis*) induces a chancre-like lesion, which is followed by enlargement of regional lymph nodes, with possibly a mild constitutional reaction. Diagnosis is established by direct demonstration of the organism in material from miliary abscesses in the border of the lesion, by culture and by specially stained biopsy specimens. The course of primary inoculation of blastomycosis is relatively benign although often prolonged.

In a second type of blastomycosis there is no history of injury and no primary lesion. The infection first appears as a nodule or papule, single or multiple, that breaks down and discharges purulent material in which the organism may be demonstrated. The lesion enlarges slowly and eccentrically, leaving a dense scar. The border is characteristic and contains miliary abscesses. The infection extends indefinitely, and little immunity develops. The treatment of choice is amphotericin B (by intravenous drip), a toxic drug that should be given only under close observation in hospital.

The variety of the disease known as South American blastomycosis, in which the infection is derived from the soil, is common among rural workers. Its course is quite different from that of North American blastomycosis, although the causative organism is very similar.

Coccidioidomycosis

This disease is acquired when spores of the organism (*Coccidioides immitis*) are inhaled from dust in certain dry areas of California, Arizona, New Mexico and Nevada. Rodents and domestic animals also become infected, but the disease is not transmitted from man to man or from animal to man.

The initial pulmonary infection of coccidioidomycosis may be symptomless, or it may produce an acute respiratory infection of varying severity. About 20 per cent of such patients develop erythema nodosum, often accompanied by arthralgia and eosinophilia.

Progression of the infection may occur in 0.1 to 1.0 per cent of white patients, but it is 5 to 10 times more frequent in blacks. Blacks should never be permitted to work in a laboratory where *C. immitis* is being grown in culture.

Dissemination of the infection may occur to any organ of the body. Except in localized forms, the disease is extremely serious, with a mortality rate of 50 per cent. Amphotericin B intravenously is being used in the treatment of the disease. Coccidioidin skin tests are of much value in epidemiologic surveys and in determining changes in the immune status of infected patients.

Sporotrichosis

This disease is caused by *Sporothrix schenckii* (formerly called *Sporotrichum schenckii*) and is an exogenous infection that is worldwide. Thousands of infections have occurred in mine workers in South Africa, and occasional cases are seen in horticulturists and agricultural workers.

The clinical course of the disease is highly characteristic. An inoculation chancre occurs at the site of injury. On the extremities, the more common site of infection, nodules develop in linear "pipestem" fashion along the lymphatics. The primary inoculation site enlarges, often with development of satellite lesions. The nodules tend to break down and suppurate rather rapidly. The organisms are demonstrable with the PAS stain and by culture. Potassium iodide in moderate doses is ordinarily curative.

Sporotrichosis may sometimes extend into underlying tissue or into organs, such as the eye, in its lymphatic pathway. Rarely does the disease become systemic by hematogenous dissemination of the organism.

Other deep fungal infections include histoplasmosis, actinomycosis, cryptococcosis, chromoblastomycosis and mycetoma (Madura foot), but, aside from histoplasmosis, in which skin lesions are rarely seen, they will seldom be encountered in general practice.

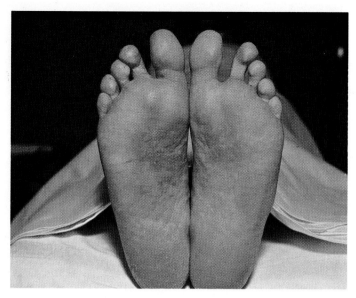

Figure 17–1.   Chronic vesicular fungal infection

This infection, caused by *Trichophyton mentagrophytes,* was subject to recurrent flare-ups from hyperhidrosis and occlusion. The diagnosis may be suspected but is not conclusive without mycologic confirmation, usually from examination of scrapings.

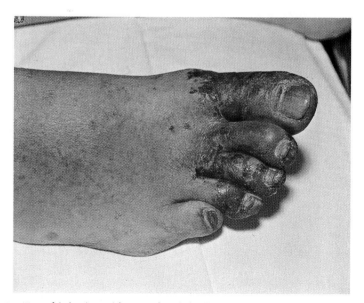

Figure 17–2.   Fungal infection with secondary infection

Irritation and secondary infection of fungal infection from over-vigorous topical medication. Note contact dermatitis of dorsum of foot.

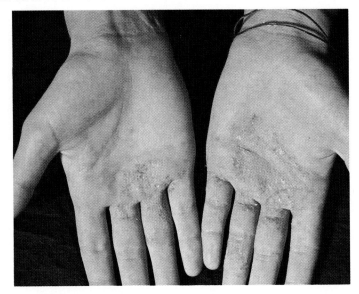

Figure 17–3.   Fungal infection of hands

Mycologic confirmation advisable. Factors other than fungi are more frequent causes of superficial inflammatory changes of the hands.

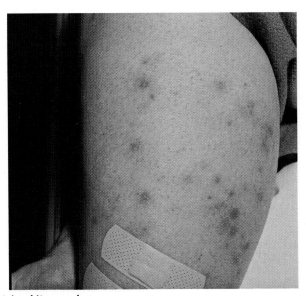

Figure 17–4.   Majocchi's granuloma

Small follicular inflamed papules of lower leg in patient with *Trichophyton rubrum* infection of feet. The follicular invasion is caused by irritation from shaving the legs.

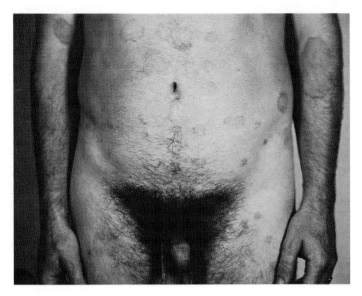

Figure 17–5.   Tinea corporis

Widespread multiple annular fungal lesions appear to mimic severe pityriasis rosea and secondary syphilis. Extensive tinea corporis is seen most frequently in the tropics. When such lesions persist in temperate climates or prove resistant to combined topical and systemic therapy, an underlying systemic disease or drug immunosuppression must be suspected.

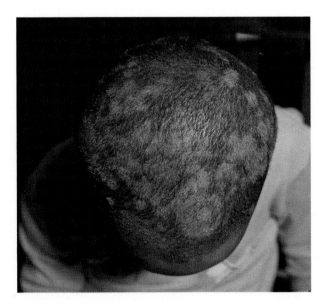

Figure 17–6.   Tinea capitis

For many years, *Microsporum audouini,* an ectothrix that fluoresces brightly under a Wood's light, produced epidemics of tinea capitis among American children in schools and other institutions. Currently, both juvenile and adult tinea capitis is most frequently produced by *Trichophyton tonsurans,* an endothrix that does *not* fluoresce under a Wood's light. A KOH preparation and culture of the involved hair is required to establish the correct diagnosis. Systemic griseofulvin therapy is the treatment of choice.

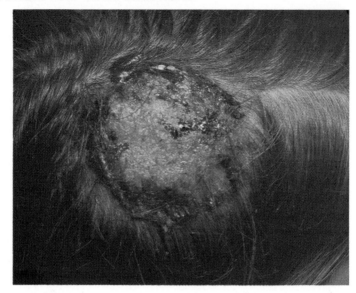

Figure 17–7.   Kerion

Boggy inflamed granuloma at site of patch of tinea capitis, due to increased sensitivity to fungi, *not* bacterial infection. Undergoes spontaneous resolution. Outlook for hair regrowth excellent.

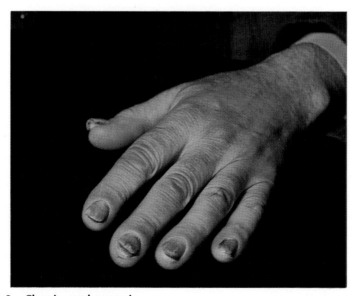

Figure 17–8.   Chronic onychomycosis

Longstanding fungal infection with secondary invasion of chromogenic bacteria. The responsible fungus may be difficult to isolate.

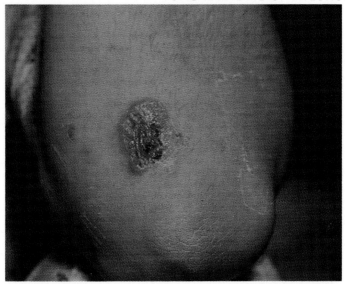

Figure 17–9.   Blastomycosis

Primary inoculation syndrome of several weeks' duration. The central ulceration and border sloping toward the periphery are well shown. Typical miliary abscesses were present. Excellent response to intravenous amphotericin B, though at risk of nephrotoxicity.

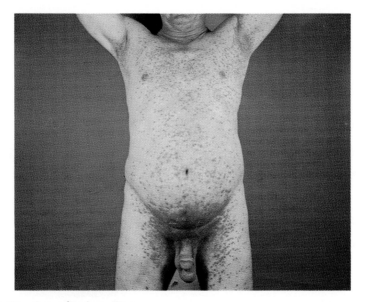

Figure 17–10.   Generalized moniliasis

Unusually extensive *Candida* infection. Note marked involvement of groin and axillae. Hot environment was a factor. Suspect systemic disease.

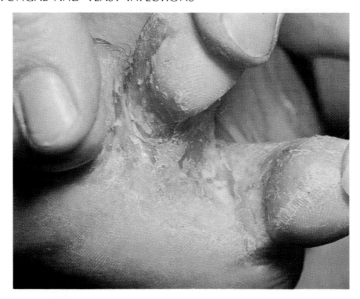

Figure 17–11.   Candidiasis (Moniliasis)

The diagnosis may be suspected on clinical examination, but examination of scales and cultures is necessary to establish it with certainty. The *Candida* may be a secondary invader. Nystatin is the preferred local treatment.

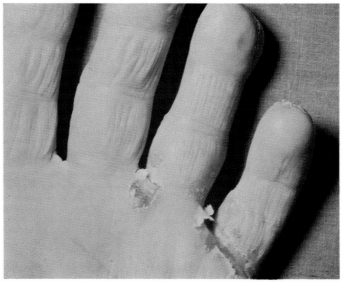

Figure 17–12.   Candidiasis (Moniliasis)

When this infection occurs on the hands, it tends to be drier and less macerated than when on the foot. Excessive exposure to water and detergents favors chronicity or recurrences.

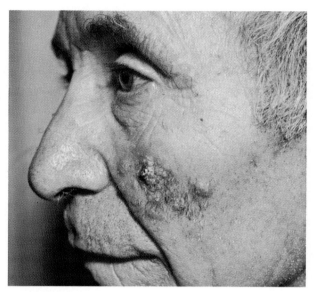

Figure 17–13.   Sporotrichosis

The infection developed after slight thorn injury sustained by gardener. Rapidly responsive to potassium iodide therapy as a rule.

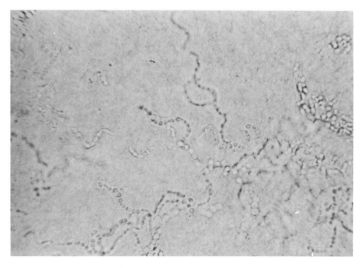

Figure 17–14.   KOH Preparation (40 ×)

Potassium hydroxide 20 per cent is added to the slide upon which have been placed scales scraped from an area suspected of containing fungi. The preparation is then viewed with a microscope, using low intensity illumination.

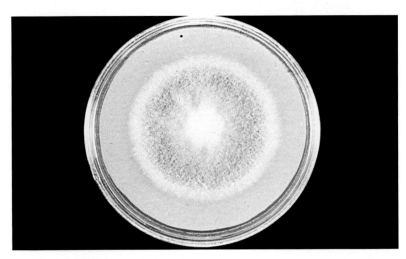

Figure 17–15. *Trichophyton rubrum* **culture**

Infected scales are placed on appropriate media (as Sabouraud's glucose agar) and grow well aerobically at room temperature. Proper identification is based upon gross colonial and microscopic morphology.

Viral and Rickettsial Infections | 18

VIRAL INFECTIONS

Certain viral infections tend to produce their most marked changes in the skin. In some, e.g., warts and molluscum, the lesions are entirely cutaneous. In another, herpes simplex, there is usually neurocutaneous involvement and a potentiality for serious systemic involvement; in others, e.g., rubeola (measles), rubella (German measles), varicella (chicken pox) or variola (smallpox), the skin lesions are only diagnostically useful expressions of the systemic infection.

Herpes Simplex (Herpes Virus Hominis — HVH)

The so-called cold sore or herpes labialis is most commonly caused by HVH Type I and is among the most frequent infectious diseases of man. The symptoms and signs are too well known to require any detailed description, because the prodromal tingling of the area and the appearance of a cluster of tense vesicles that eventuate in a crust have been experienced by a high percentage of the adult population. At times, the lesions of herpes simplex may be quite large, covering an area of 2 cm. or more in diameter. The discomfort and swelling may be marked.

It is to be kept in mind that herpes simplex lesions may occur on any part of the skin surface. When they occur on the genitalia, they are known as herpes progenitalis and are most commonly caused by HVH Type II. In females with recurrent HVH Type II vaginal infection, there appears to be an increased incidence of carcinoma of the cervix, a most important epidemiologic correlation.

The initial infection with herpes simplex may occur in infants or young children as pharyngostomatitis. The local inflammatory changes may be very marked and the systemic signs grave. Occasionally, the outcome is fatal. This severe primary herpetic infection may occasionally be seen in adult life, most frequently as vulvovaginitis. Systemic and disseminated cutaneous infection by the herpes simplex virus may be a

259

serious complication of atopic dermatitis. (Herpetic meningitis is an uncommon complication but a most serious one.

Herpes near the eye requires the greatest concern, because involvement of the eye has serious implications. In herpes involving the conjunctiva or surrounding skin, ophthalmologic consultation is mandatory.

Though the common term "cold sore" indicates that herpes simplex is most frequently associated with an upper respiratory infection or febrile illness, there are other precipitating factors that are no less important. Some individuals regularly develop herpes simplex with exposure to sunlight. Recurrence in relation to the menses is common. There is some indication that exhaustion and stress may play a role. As a rule, the lesions tend to occur in almost precisely the same spot.

It is not uncommon for herpes simplex to involve the finger in individuals who perform oral examinations, such as physicians, dentists or nurses. It manifests itself as a painful, tense group of vesicles, usually of the distal phalanx. Regional lymphadenopathy is common. Differentiation from a bacterial infection is aided by the demonstration of multinucleated giant cells from the base of a vesicle.

Prevention and Treatment.   There is no regularly satisfactory method of preventing recurrences of herpes simplex. If specific precipitating factors can be determined, these should be avoided. Repeated vaccination with smallpox vaccine has been widely used, but its effectiveness as a preventive agent is uncertain.

The treatment of herpes simplex affecting the skin is likewise unsatisfactory. Spirits of camphor or 10 per cent camphor in alcohol may assist in drying up the lesion. *Corticosteroid preparations are strongly contraindicated* in acute herpes involving the eye or surrounding skin. Idoxuridine is helpful in herpes simplex of the eye, but not in skin infections. Photoactive dye therapy is not recommended. Patients with light-activated lesions should use sunscreens on a routine basis, especially during the summertime.

Zoster (Herpes Zoster, Shingles)

This highly characteristic eruption is caused by the same virus (VZ) that produces varicella (chickenpox). Adults who develop zoster almost always give a history of having had varicella in childhood. There is reasonable evidence to indicate that the virus has been dormant since the original episode of varicella and then produces a recurrence in a different form. Zoster, however, apparently may be exogenously acquired.

Zoster is almost invariably unilateral and occurs in a distribution pattern that corresponds to that of a ganglion or ganglia within the central nervous system. The most common type is that occurring on the trunk, but any area of the body may be involved, including the face and lower extremities. In these areas the diagnosis is not infrequently missed. The lesions consist of groups of tense vesicles on an erythematous base, sometimes few in number, but not infrequently coalescent along a linear area. The duration of the inflammation varies, but there is a general correlation of the severity of the local changes and pain with the age of the patient. In children, zoster may produce no pain at all, and the lesions may be relatively evanescent over a period of 10 days to 2 weeks. In elderly patients or in persons with significant systemic disease, such as uncontrolled diabetes or lymphoma, the local lesions may be exceedingly severe, even to the point of necrosis, and the neuralgic pain almost unbearable.

The appearance of the eruption is ordinarily heralded by tingling or pain in the affected areas 2 or more days prior to the onset of the lesions. Marked pain from the beginning is worrisome in respect to the development of "postherpetic neuralgia," which may persist for months or years after the eruption has subsided. Children with leukemia or on long-term corticosteroid therapy are extremely vulnerable to the virus of zoster. The same applies to patients who are immunosuppressed by disease or medications.

Zoster involving the gasserian ganglion and the ophthalmic branch of the trigeminal nerve is of serious portent in respect to involvement of the eye. Ophthalmologic consultation is always indicated.

Although no precise figures are available, the relatively common occurrence of zoster in patients with known malignant disease is striking. In such individuals, particularly those with a lymphoma, the zoster may be accompanied by a sparse or profuse generalized varicelliform eruption that is indistinguishable from ordinary chickenpox and is indeed the same disease. This may sometimes occur in otherwise healthy individuals.

The treatment of zoster will be dependent upon the severity of the local changes and the symptoms. In mild zoster nothing more than the local application of a drying lotion is indicated. In severe zoster, particularly in the ophthalmic type, systemic steroid therapy is indicated. Some observers favor the administration of ACTH intravenously, but this has given way to oral doses of prednisone or its equivalent, initially given in doses of 40 to 60 mg. daily. Measures to ease the pain are often necessary, but addiction-inducing drugs should be avoided if possible. The course of steroid therapy ordinarily need not be a prolonged one. Such therapy does not appear to shorten the course of zoster but unquestionably reduces the severity of pain and local inflammatory effects. In severe single lesions, the injection of a solution of a corticosteroid and lidocaine (Xylocaine) may be helpful.

Warts

Warts represent an extremely common banal tumor due to a virus, for which there is no really satisfactory treatment. The treatment of an undoubted viral infection by surgical or cauterant chemotherapeutic methods is medieval, but no effective antiviral compound is available. A wart may persist as a single lesion for many years and then disappear without treatment, or there may be multiple lesions. The most troublesome warts are those involving a pressure surface on the sole or the paronychial margins. Unfortunately, in both of these areas, treatment may be unsuccessful. Warts vary greatly in their appearance. The most common type is a slightly raised papule with a dry grayish rough surface. In the perianal region warts are often large, moist and exuberant, with a whitish color (venereal warts). On the face, warts are often small, flat and brownish in color. Plantar warts are not usually raised much above the surface because they are surrounded by a marked protective thickening of the stratum corneum.

Treatment. In evaluating the effectiveness of any type of treatment of warts it must be kept in mind that these lesions may disappear spontaneously and are sometimes susceptible to psychotherapy. If one or two or three warts are not bothersome or conspicuous, it is sometimes best to let them alone.

Electrodesiccation. If there are only a few warts, probably the best way to remove them is by electrodesiccation and gentle curettage under local anesthesia. After the lesion is softened with conservative electrodesiccation, it is curetted off and the bleeding points controlled with light desiccation. There is no advantage, indeed there is considerable disadvantage, in carrying the electrodesiccation more deeply. Following the removal of the average wart, there should be either no scar whatever or a very minimal one. *This method should not be used on weight-bearing surfaces of the soles.* On this thick surface, scarring may be inevitable, and the scar, particularly if it is over the head of a metatarsal, is often worse symptomatically than the original wart. Simple curettage under local anesthesia is sometimes effective in plantar warts, but *without electrodesiccation.* Full thickness surgical excision of a plantar wart on a weight-bearing surface is almost always followed by a painful scar.

One of the most common mistakes in the management of painful plantar lesions is failure to differentiate between a scar and a true wart. A scar on the sole is hard and keratinous throughout, while a wart is soft and whitish at the base.

Other methods of treatment are legion. A few will be listed here.

Liquid Nitrogen. If this material is available, it offers a reasonably satisfactory, relatively nontechnical method of treating warts. Freezing is induced by applying liquid nitrogen with a cotton applicator intermittently for a period of 20 to 30 seconds The reaction that follows varies, but if a blister forms, the wart is frequently lifted off with it. Caution should be used not to overdo the method in treating plantar warts. Several treatments may be necessary.

Salicylic Acid Plaster. This method may be tried by applying a 35 per cent plaster, allowing it to remain for 2 days and then curetting or soaking off the softened tissue. The effectiveness may be increased by the preliminary application of phenol and fuming nitric acid.

TRICHLORACETIC OR DICHLORACETIC ACID.   These have long been used for the treatment of warts, but the results are far from spectacular. It should be kept in mind that this material is *extremely dangerous in the hands of children.* A completely unnecessary, agonizing tragedy may result.

PODOPHYLLIN.   A sometimes useful method of treating plantar warts is the application of 20 per cent podophyllin in compound tincture of benzoin every other day, followed by the application of occlusive adhesive tape. *Caution: Podophyllin is extremely injurious to the eyes.* It is most effective in moist "venereal" warts. In such warts, to prevent undue reaction, the patient should sit in a tub bath 3 to 4 hours after application. Occlusion is not necessary. Occasional sensitization reactions may be encountered. In intertrigenous areas, secondary infection may be a complication.

X-ray therapy of plantar warts is still used by some physicians. The dose should be low enough so that it does not produce atrophy.

Molluscum Contagiosum

Molluscum contagiosum is caused by a pox virus. The clinical appearance of the lesions produced by it are highly characteristic, and the diagnosis is easily confirmed by the demonstration of molluscum bodies in stained smears of the crumbly semisolid material expressed from the lesions.

The lesions of molluscum contagiosum are yellowish, raised papules, 2 to 5 mm. in diameter, with a characteristic dell at the summit of the lesion. They may be few or multiple. Occasionally they reach the size of a centimeter or more (giant molluscum). Inflammation of the base may develop, giving the appearance of a low grade furuncle. Such lesions may involute spontaneously.

Treatment.   This is simple; all that is necessary is to extrude the lesion with a Schamberg comedone extractor or with a pointed applicator stick, a procedure sometimes objected to rather vociferously by young children. Considerable slow bleeding from the base may be encountered, but this is easily controlled by pressure. The procedure produces no scarring. Application of a drop of tricloracetic acid to the central dell of the lesion is sometimes curative. Treatment by electrodesiccation is unnecessary and unduly destructive.

Infectious Exanthemata

Exanthema Subitum (Roseola).   This is a fairly common exanthematous disease in children of ages 6 to 18 months. It is probably viral in origin. It is characterized by a sudden onset with fever. This may persist for as long as 5 days but subsides with the appearance of the exanthem.

The eruption is macular and usually appears first on the trunk, with little involvement of the face or the distal portion of the extremities. It may be distinguished from measles by the absence of Koplik spots. The relative absence of lymphadenitis and the subsidence of fever with the appearance of the eruption distinguish it from German measles.

Measles (Rubeola).   This myxoviral infection is endemic throughout the world, but the increasing extension of vaccination programs promises to reduce its incidence greatly. The chief features of the disease are (1) a prodrome developing some 7 days after exposure, consisting of fever, conjunctivitis, occasional severe photophobia and a running nose; (2) the appearance of Koplik spots in the mouth, small bluish white lesions 1 to 2 mm. in diameter, usually around the orifice of the parotid duct and sometimes on the lower lip; and (3) a macular or maculopapular eruption, appearing first on the forehead and behind the ears and then spreading over the face, trunk and extremities.

Measles is highly infectious during the prodromal phase and for a few days after the appearance of the eruption. In exposed individuals, particularly sickly children or nonimmune adults, the administration of gamma globulin in a dose of 0.2 to 0.3 ml. per kg. body weight on the first to eighth day of incubation furnishes protection, but if the disease is aborted, immunity does not develop.

Secondary trailing bacterial infection and, uncommonly, severe encephalitis are the chief complications of measles.

German Measles (Rubella).   This viral infection is of relatively little importance to the patient but of major risk to the fetus of a pregnant woman who acquires the disease during the first trimester of pregnancy. There is a 50 to 80 per cent chance of early or delayed fetal malformations, principally deafness, microencephaly, cardiac malformations, dental abnormalities and ophthalmologic defects.

The rash of German measles appears as round pink macules that may sometimes be so confluent as to resemble scarlet fever. It ordinarily develops on the head and reaches full extension over the trunk within 24 hours. It persists for only 2 or 3 days. *Cervical and occipital lymphadenopathy* are characteristic, and *there are no Koplik spots* as in measles. The rash of rubella may be simulated by that associated with Echo viral infections.

The wide extension of effective vaccination programs against German measles promises to make it an uncommon disease.

Chickenpox (Varicella).   This viral disease has the most distinctive clinical characteristics of all the infectious exanthemata. The virus is the same as that of herpes zoster. The principal features of chickenpox are as follows: (1) an incubation period averaging 2 weeks, (2) mild prodromal symptoms of slight fever and malaise, (3) tense clear vesicles on an erythematous base, continuing to appear over a period of several days, (4) distribution principally to the trunk and face, but no lesions on palms and soles (as in smallpox), (5) mucous membrane lesions appearing as small vesicles that rapidly become punctate ulcers and (6) evolution of skin lesions with characteristic brownish crusts, with healing within a week or so, unless complicated by bacterial infection (uncommon) or repeated picking off of the crusts, resulting in increased scarring.

The infection may be severe, even lethal, in neonatal infants, in children on long-term corticosteroid therapy or in patients with leukemia. Meningoencephalitis is rare. Varicella pneumonia may occur.

TREATMENT. Little therapy is indicated in the average case. Drying topical preparations, rather than ointments, should be used. Secondary bacterial infection should be dealt with systemically. The patient should be admonished not to pick off the crusts, an urge that is sometimes uncontrollable.

Smallpox (Variola). The average physician in the United States, Britain, continental Europe or the USSR will probably never see a case of smallpox in his professional lifetime. Nevertheless, because isolated epidemics continue to occur occasionally, consideration of the disease should not be allowed to sink completely below the diagnostic horizon.

The chief diagnostic features of variola are (1) a suddenly developing prodrome of headache, backache, high fever, chills and malaise, (2) appearance of the exanthem in 3 or 4 days in the form of papules distributed chiefly to the face and extremities and *involving the palms and soles* (a distinguishing feature from varicella), (3) appearance of the lesions all at once, not in crops as in varicella and (4) progression of the lesions through vesicles and pustules, with crusting within 2 weeks.

Smallpox does not follow the classic course in partially immunized persons, and the diagnosis may be missed in the initial patient(s), becoming apparent only when secondary contacts develop the disease. This occurred in New York City in 1947.

Practical diagnostic virologic methods are available.

RICKETTSIAL INFECTIONS

Rickettsiae are small pleomorphic obligate intracellular microorganisms. They take the form of short rods or cocci, exist singly, in pairs, in short chains or in filaments and live symbiotically with arthropods. In their natural hosts they may be passed on to new generations of hosts transovarially. In an unnatural host, such as man, they may produce disease. The organisms invade endothelial cells and the smooth muscle cells surrounding small blood vessels. As the organisms multiply, the vessel lumens become occluded and may rupture, producing purpuric lesions in the skin, brain or other body organs.

The diagnosis of rickettsial disease depends in large part upon a high index of suspicion and suggestive clinical findings. Serologic testing and embryonated egg cultures serve as confirmatory tests but are not of immediate diagnostic help early in the course of the infection.

The therapy of choice is a tetracycline given in a dose of 2 to 3 gm. daily. In early cases, response to therapy should be seen within 24 to 48 hours. Therapy should be continued 5 to 7 days beyond the initial response. In resistant or well-established infections, chloramphenicol 2 to 3 gm. per day might be considered as an alternative drug. Pancytopenia may result from the use of chloramphenicol, so it must be used with caution. Sulfonamides are contraindicated, since they consistently enhance rickettsial disease.

The following is a brief summary of the principal rickettsial infections. It is unlikely that, with the exception of Rocky Mountain spotted fever, any of these will be seen in general practice. Others, however, may become widely epidemic in pediculous populations. In Naples, Italy, for instance, a foreboding outbreak occurred in 1943 to 1944, constituting a threat to the population and large numbers of Allied troops in the area. The outbreak was promptly controlled by DDT dusting of the entire population, civilian and military.

Typhus

Epidemic Typhus. This rickettsial infection is transmitted by body lice, occasionally by head lice. The causative organism is *Rickettsia prowazekii*. The organism is found in large numbers in the louse feces. The initial signs are headache, chills, generalized pain and weakness. A macular rash appears, first on the trunk, then spreads, exempting the face, palms and soles. Frank hemorrhagic changes may develop, a serious prognostic sign.

Overwhelming toxicity develops in untreated cases, involving the myocardium, bone marrow, spleen, kidneys and lungs. Treatment consists of broad spectrum antibiotics in large doses, justifiable even before the diagnosis is established precisely. Epidemiologic consultation is imperative.

Detection of louse infestation in the general population and prompt control of it are of the utmost importance. DDT powder is effective and nontoxic. It is, however, no longer available in the United States, having shown toxicity when incorporated in creams and ointments.

Serologic studies of suspected cases should be undertaken promptly, although the availability of facilities for such studies varies in different areas. The agglutination test using *Proteus* OX-19 is the most generally employed, but it does not become significantly positive until 5 or more days after onset of the infection.

Murine Typhus. This infection is difficult to differentiate from epidemic typhus, the clinical feature being involvement of the face, palms and soles. In addition to man, the animal hosts in murine typhus may include rats, mice and squirrels. Control is achieved by the elimination of these vectors, along with the application of DDT powder to the population at risk. Broad spectrum antibiotics offer effective treatment.

Spotted Fever (Rocky Mountain Spotted Fever)

This rickettsial infection, caused by *R. rickettsiae* (named after the martyr Howard Taylor Ricketts, who discovered the disease and died from it), is by no means uncommon in wooded and grassy areas of North and South America during the "tick season" of warm summer months. Rural inhabitants of these areas have a healthy respect for tick bites. (Among golfers in deep rough, it might be called a "lost ball" infestation.) The tick attaches itself firmly to the skin and becomes engorged with blood. Protection is afforded by snug clothing, particulary at the ankles and wrists, but this is not particularly acceptable in warm weather. Insect repellents are indifferently effective in preventing bites. The best protection from infection is careful inspection after exposure, with particular attention to hairy areas and the male genitalia. Removal of the ticks may be accomplished in many ways. A smoldering match head usually causes it to release its grip. With manual removal, care should be taken not to contaminate the skin with the bloody contents of the tick sack. Forceps removal should be done gently in an effort to remove the embedded portion of the tick.

Untreated spotted fever is a lethal disease. Its onset is characterized by prostration and chills, usually severe. Neurologic signs are often prominent. The telltale "spotted" rash appears between the third and seventh days, usually first about the wrists and ankles, and then becomes generalized. The lesions become purpuric and very intense. As soon as the diagnosis is suspected, often on the basis of a tick bite, treatment with large doses of an antibiotic, tetracycline or chloramphenicol, is indicated. Time is of the essence.

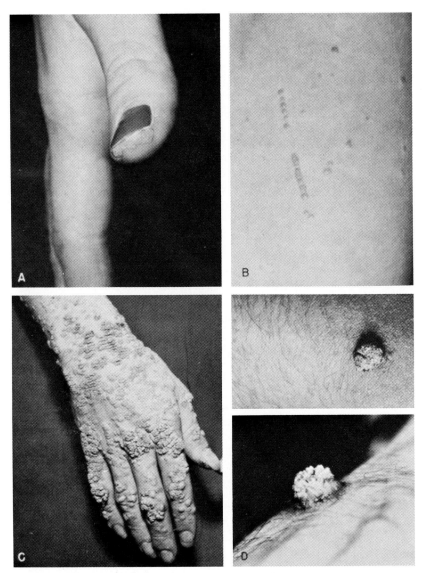

Figure 18–1.   Various types of warts

A. Periungual warts. Sometimes incurable. *B.* Inoculation of flat warts along scratch. *C.* Diffuse warts of many years duration—an insoluble therapeutic problem. *D.* Variations in size and surface of warts.

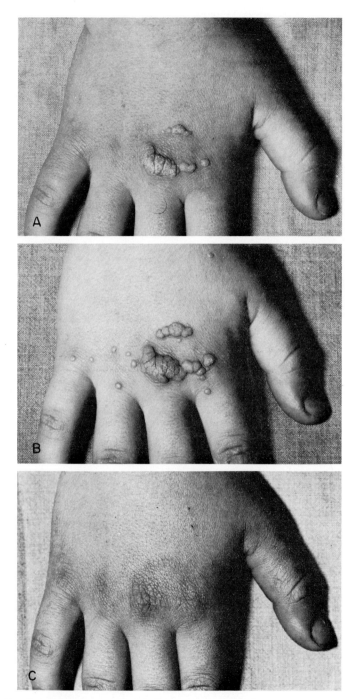

Figure 18–2. Development, spread and disappearance of warts

A. Warts in 5-year-old boy that appeared in area of superficial circular burn. The patient's mother had warts on the hands. Suggestion therapy was given. B. Six months later. Enlargement of old lesions; appearance of new ones. A grenz ray exposure (300r) was administered to the large central group only. The lesions began to disappear within three weeks. C. Eight months later. Disappearance due to suggestion(?), normal course(?) or grenz ray therapy (??).

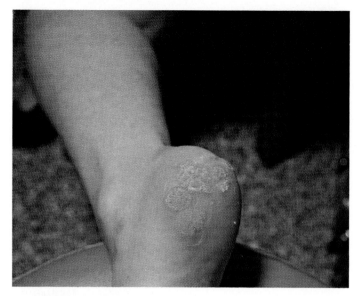

Figure 18–3. Mosaic plantar warts

After a prolonged series of chemotherapeutic procedures, cure was obtained by thorough curettage under local anesthesia, *without electrodesiccation.* A few days of bed rest are necessary, but the procedure is not unduly disabling.

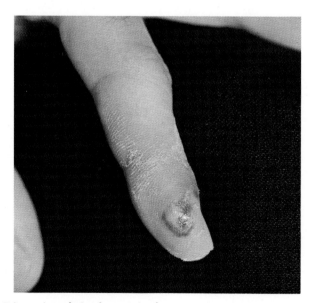

Figure 18–4. Primary inoculation herpes simplex

Occurring in a physician engaged in bare-handed oral examinations. Regional lymphadenopathy, slow healing. (Courtesy of Dr. George W. Hambrick, Jr.)

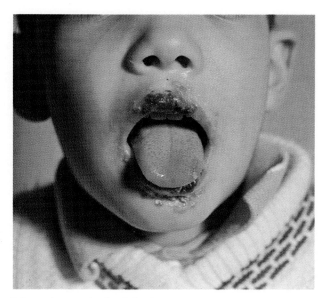

Figure 18–5.   Primary herpes simplex infection

This type is seen in children with no prior immunity to HVH. The oral lesions are severe, and the systemic manifestations may be marked. The vulva and vagina may be involved in females.

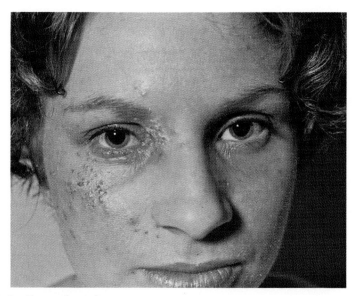

Figure 18–6.   Eczema herpeticum

Occurring in patient with atopic dermatitis and a history of contact with individual with herpes simplex. The involvement around the eye is worrisome. *Topical corticosteroid therapy absolutely contraindicated.*

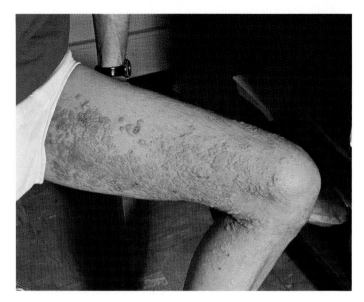

Figure 18–7. Zoster

Severe herpes zoster in a patient with Hodgkin's disease. Note the purpuric elements in some lesions. In extensive painful cases, short-term corticosteroid therapy may be indicated. Intralesional steroids (not to exceed triamcinolone acetonide 2 mgm./cc.) may be helpful in minimizing pain and tissue destruction in small localized skin lesions. In immunosuppressed patients, herpes zoster may evolve into a generalized viremia with a varicelliform eruption as well as other organ system involvement.

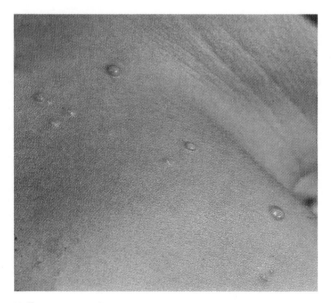

Figure 18–8. Molluscum contagiosum

Multiple small papules. Shiny, light yellow color. Characteristic dell at summit. Cured by expression of contents as for large comedone.

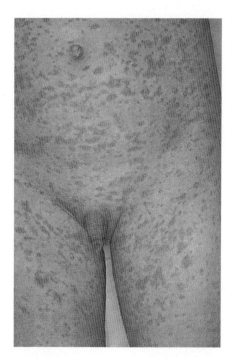

Figure 18–9. Measles

(Used by permission from Korting, G. W., Diseases of the Skin in Children and Adolescents. W. B. Saunders Co., 1970.)

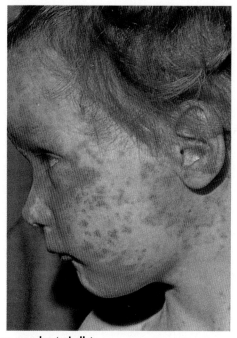

Figure 18–10. German measles (rubella)

(Used by permission from Korting, G. W., Diseases of the Skin in Children and Adolescents. W. B. Saunders Co., 1970.)

273

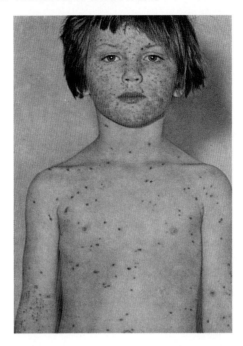

Figure 18–11. Varicella (chickenpox) resembling navigational chart of the stars

(Used by permission from Korting, G. W.; Diseases of the Skin in Children and Adolescents. W. B. Saunders Co., 1970.)

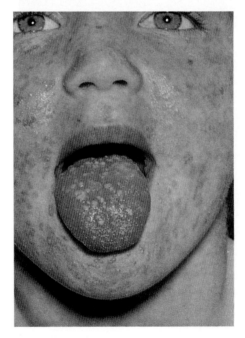

Figure 18–12. Chickenpox lesions on the tongue

(Used by permission from Korting, G. W., Diseases of the Skin in Children and Adolescents. W. B. Saunders Co., 1970.)

19

Syphilis, Chancroid, Lymphogranuloma Venereum and Granuloma Inguinale

In this chapter, the cutaneous and mucous membrane signs of syphilis, chancroid, lymphogranuloma venereum and granuloma inguinale will be reviewed. Currently accepted confirmatory laboratory methods, treatment schedules and follow-up procedures will be included.

SYPHILIS

Following the introduction and widespread use of penicillin in the treatment of syphilis in 1942 to 1943, a steady decline in syphilis cases was noted in the United States and all parts of the civilized world. This trend was reversed in the latter 1950's in the United States, and early syphilis remains a significant health problem. Late syphilis, so frequently seen in prepenicillin days in the form of aortic aneurysm, tabes dorsalis, paresis, skin gummas and other distinctive lesions, has become a medical rarity.

The course and characteristics of early syphilis are as follows.

The Chancre (Primary Syphilis). A hard, button-like eroded lesion of the penis occurs from 2 to 10 weeks after exposure. A similar lesion occurs in the vagina, but it is not commonly observed and diagnosed.

With the chancre, indurated, enlarged, nontender, nonfluctuant regional lymph nodes develop. In a chancre located elsewhere than on the genitalia, e.g., the lips, the associated lymph node enlargement (bubo) is ordinarily very great. The possibility of extragenital chancres on the lips or anus is particularly high in homosexuals and in heterosexuals indulging in oral-genital contacts.

DIAGNOSIS. *Darkfield examination* of serum obtained from the chancre is used to demonstrate the *Treponema pallidum*. Unfortunately, the number of physicians and technicians capable of performing this procedure expertly is much less than when syphilis was more prevalent. Lesions in the mouth and at the anal orifice are untrustworthy sources of serum for darkfield examination because they may yield spirochetes that are indistinguishable from *T. pallidum*.

Secondary Syphilis. In this stage, which develops 6 or more weeks after the appearance of the chancre, lesions may develop anywhere in the body as a result of dissemination of treponemata throughout the blood stream. The organs most commonly involved are the skin and mucous membranes. The most characteristic lesions are:

1. Eroded painless patches of the mouth or vagina (mucous patches)

2. White, moist, wart-like lesions of the perianal region

3. Circinate, pigmented papular lesions of the face

4. Flat, hard, slightly scaling papules of the hands and soles.

5. A faint roseola eruption of the trunk. In late secondary syphilis the lesions are distinctly papular or papulo-pustular. Vesicular-bullous lesions are not seen in acquired lesions in adults.

6. A patchy, moth-eaten-appearing partial alopecia of the occipital and temple portions of the scalp

7. Generalized nontender lymphadenopathy

The open lesions of secondary syphilis are highly infectious. Individuals exposed to them should receive appropriate prophylactic antibiotic therapy to prevent the development of early syphilis.

Visceral involvement may occur in secondary syphilis. Although uncommon, iritis, iridocyclitis, periostitis, lytic lesions of the long bones, nephritis and meningitis may occur. Response to penicillin therapy is usually rapid, and permanent pathological changes are rare.

Treatment

Early Syphilis. Currently accepted treatment schedules for primary syphilis, secondary syphilis and latent syphilis of less than a year's duration are:

1. Benzathine penicillin G, 2.4 million units total by a single intramuscular injection or

2. Aqueous procaine penicillin G, 4.8 million units total: 600,000 units by intramuscular injection daily for 8 days.

PATIENTS WHO ARE ALLERGIC TO PENICILLIN MAY BE TREATED WITH

1. Tetracycline hydrochloride, 500 mg., 4 times daily by mouth for 15 days or

2. Erythromycin (sterate, ethylsuccinate or base), 500 mg., 4 times a day by mouth for 15 days.*

---

*Venereal Disease Control Advisory Committee: Syphilis: Recommended treatment schedules. Ann. of Intern. Med. *85*(1):94–96, 1976.

The early signs of a penicillin reaction are itching, vertigo, flushing and urticaria. Hoarseness may develop along with precipitous hypotension. Epinephrine (0.5 cc. of 1:1000 solution intramuscularly) should be given along with 100 mg. hydrocortisone intravenously. Oxygen and cardiopulmonary resuscitation measures may be necessary. In any severe reaction to penicillin, treatment within minutes is of critical importance in saving the patient's life.

The Herxheimer reaction occurs within 12 hours after the injection of penicillin in a high percentage of patients with early syphilis. This consists of headache, malaise, fever and chills. It should not be confused with a reaction to penicillin.

Late Syphilis. For the currently accepted treatment schedules of late latent syphilis, late manifest syphilis, congenital syphilis and syphilis of pregnancy, the reader is referred to the volume 85 issue of *Annals of Internal Medicine* (July, 1976), pages 94 to 96.

Serologic Tests for Syphilis (STS)

Two groups of serologic tests, the cardiolipin and treponemal, are available for the diagnosis and follow-up of the treponemal diseases of man — syphilis, yaws, pinta and bejel. Generally, the serologic principles described for syphilis apply to the other diseases. In any event, none of the serologic tests may be used to differentiate between the four treponematoses.

Cardiolipin Tests. These are screening tests for syphilis. The rapid plasma reagin (RPR) test, automated reagin test (ART) and Venereal Disease Research Laboratories (VDRL) test are common examples of this group. Their primary functions are to alert the clinician to the possibility of a treponemal infection and to serve as a barometer of the adequacy of therapy. In early syphilis (of less than 1 year's duration), a rapidly rising titer is virtually diagnostic of an *active* infection. Similarly, a falling titer usually indicates adequate therapy. In the cerebrospinal fluid (CSF), these tests are widely used to detect the presence of syphilitic antibody.

Treponemal Tests. These tests are confirmatory. The fluorescent treponemal antibody absorption (FTA-ABS) test and its modifications (FTA-IgA, -IgG and -IgM), as well as the *Treponema pallidum* immobilization (TPI) test, are used to confirm the presence of treponemal antibodies in the serum of patients with reactive cardiolipin tests. They are *not* valuable in determining the activity of disease or the adequacy of treatment. They tend to remain reactive indefinitely.

False-Positive Tests. Biologic false-positive (BFP) tests for syphilis occur with connective tissue diseases to produce chronic, or long-term, false-positive tests and with acute processes, such as drug eruptions, viremias (cowpox, primary herpes simplex and infectious mononucleosis) and bacterial infections (tuberculosis, leprosy and pneumococcal pneumonia) to produce short-term, or acute, false-positive tests. The false-positive tests seen in pregnancy, thyroiditis and immune-complex disorders are best described as chronic false-positive tests. Test results are designated as chronic if they persist for more than 6 months after removal or control of inciting agents. In most cases, only the cardiolipin tests have false-positive reactions. Recently, however, false-positive treponemal tests have been reported to be associated with tumors of the central nervous system,* drug eruptions and the collagen diseases. It is therefore important to carefully evaluate the patient in the light of clinical findings and epidemiologic history. Blind serologic data may be very misleading.

CHANCROID

This ulcerative venereal disease occurs in the genital area within 3 to 5 days after exposure, an incubation period much less than that of syphilis. The initial lesion is ordinarily a small pustule that breaks down to form a tender, often painful, ulcer. Unlike the chancre of syphilis, the lesions of chancroid are frequently multiple. The destructiveness of the lesion varies greatly, but if untreated, an extending deep ulcer may result and may persist for months. Fluctuant buboes in the area of drainage are the rule.

Laboratory confirmation of the diagnosis of chancroid may be difficult. The demonstration of small gram-negative rods in the base of ulcers or in bubo aspirates is helpful. *Hemophilus ducreyi* may be grown on eosin methylene blue (EMB) blood agar or, in some cases, on a clot from the patient's blood that has been inoculated with bubo aspirate.

To facilitate diagnostic accuracy, primary and recurrent herpes simplex infections should be excluded with a Tzank smear for viral giant cells; syphilis should be excluded by 3 consecutive negative darkfield examinations, a nonreactive cardiolipin test (e.g., RPR or VDRL) and a nonreactive treponemal test (e.g., FTA-ABS).

Treatment

The treatment of chancroid should include both topical and systemic therapy.

Topical. Therapy should include careful cleansing of the affected area 3 to 4 times a day with a nonirritating antibacterial soap to prevent autoinoculation of the surrounding skin. Repeated aspiration of fluctuant buboes is necessary in order to prevent spontaneous rupture and sinus tract formation. Wide surgical incisions is inadvisable.

Systemic. Therapy for chancroid has undergone some re-evaluation

---

*Delaney, P.: False positive serology in cerebrospinal fluid associated with a spinal cord tumor. Neurology 26:591–593, 1976.

in the last few years because antibiotic-resistant strains have begun to emerge in various areas of the world — particularly in the Far East. In descending order of preference, the following systemic treatment regimens are suggested:

1. SULFISOXAZOLE. One gram every 6 hours by mouth, combined with *tetracycline hydrochloride,* 500 mg. by mouth every 6 hours for at least 14 days or until all lesions have completely healed. Some patients require up to 28 days of the *combined* therapy for total resolution of skin and bubo lesions.

2. SULFISOXAZOLE. One gram every 6 hours by mouth for at least 14 days or until all lesions have completely cleared. If there is, however, no evidence of clinical healing after 7 days of therapy, the possibility of a drug-resistant organism must be considered. Tetracycline hydrochloride should be added to the regimen (regimen 1), or other alternative antibiotics should be considered.

3. TETRACYCLINE HYDROCHLORIDE. This drug (or other tetracycline derivatives) may be used alone if the patient is allergic to sulfisoxazole. *Caution:* Therapeutic failure rates in excess of 70 per cent may be expected when using one of this group of antibiotics alone. The dosage is 500 mg. by mouth every 6 hours for at least 14 days or until all lesions have cleared. Intramuscular tetracyclines are not desirable alternatives. If there is no evidence of healing after 7 days of treatment, the possibility of a tetracycline-resistant organism must be considered and an alternative antibiotic, such as kanamycin sulfate, cephalothin sodium or chloramphenicol, considered.

Since all the principal antibiotics used in the treatment of chancroid have potentially significant side effects, a review of the pharmacology of each drug is recommended before treatment is instituted.

LYMPHOGRANULOMA VENEREUM (LGV)

This disease, although not common, may be confused with other venereal diseases. It is caused by *Chlamydia trachomatis,* serotypes L-1, L-2 and L-3. The small transitory primary lesion occurs from 1 to 3 weeks after exposure. It frequently is unnoticed, and the first indication of trouble is an inguinal bubo, which may be bilateral.

Constitutional symptoms may be noted at this time in the form of fever, chills, headache and other evidence of infection. Untreated, the infection follows lymphatic channels and may eventuate in severe proctitis, rectal stricture and multiple ulcers of the skin. In advanced untreated cases, hypertrophic longitudinal folds develop in the rectum and the sigmoid and descending colons. These may be clearly seen after barium enema.

An initial STS should be obtained and a darkfield examination done if the primary lesion is present. Serum complement fixation titers for LGV are helpful in establishing the presence of active disease and the effectiveness of treatment. Pre-and post-treatment titers are especially useful.

Treatment

Tetracycline should be given in doses of 500 mg., 4 times daily for 2 weeks, then 250 mg., 4 times daily for 2 weeks.

GRANULOMA INGUINALE

This uncommon chronic ulcerative granulomatous process is seen most frequently in multiparous women with poor perineal hygiene. It is caused by *Donovania granulomatis* and may affect the mucous membranes of the anogenital area, mouth and nasopharynx. Rarely the organisms may spread along lymphatics and produce massive inflammatory granulomas throughout the viscera. Neglected long-standing cases may undergo malignant degeneration. Recurrent secondary infection with sepsis occurs in extensive lesions or in lesions involving the vagina, cervix or urinary bladder. The diagnosis is usually confirmed by demonstrating intracytoplasmic bipolar (safety pin-like) organisms on tissue *smear* that is stained with Giemsa or Wright's stain. Silver stains of biopsy material may also be used to identify the organisms.

Treatment

Classically, streptomycin 1.0 gm. intramuscularly for 7 to 14 days produces prompt recovery in most patients. The ototoxicity of this drug, as well as the tendency of the organism to rapidly develop resistance, makes it a second line drug today. Tetracycline hydrochloride, 500 mg. 4 times a day for 3 to 4 weeks is now the treatment of choice. In tetracycline-resistant cases, ampicillin 500 mg. 4 times a day for 3 to 4 weeks is often effective.

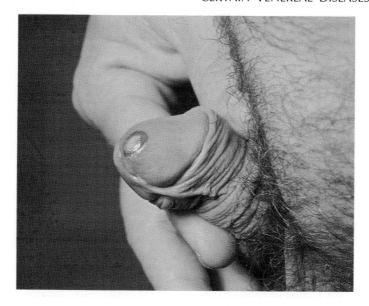

Figure 19–1.   Chancre of syphilis

The diagnosis may, of course, be suspected from the indurated eroded lesion and associated adenopathy, but it cannot be made with certainty in the absence of darkfield demonstration of *T. pallidum* or serologic confirmation.

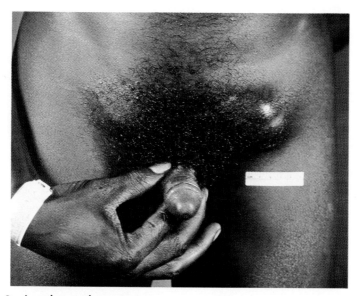

Figure 19–2.   Lymphogranuloma venereum

The portal of entry is characterized by a relatively inconspicuous and evanescent lesion, with a large fluctuant suppurative bubo. Characteristically bubos lie above and below the inguinal ligament. Note the "crease" in this patient.

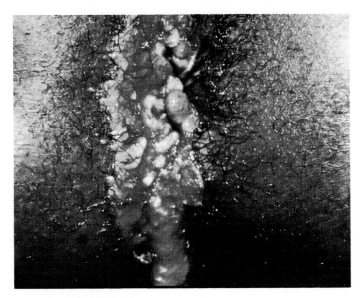

Figure 19–3. Granuloma inguinale

A now uncommon chronic ulcerative granulomatous ulcerative process caused by *Donovania granulomatis*. Diagnosis confirmable by demonstration of Donovan bodies in Giemsa stained smear. Curable with full doses of a broad spectrum antibiotic over a period of 30 days.

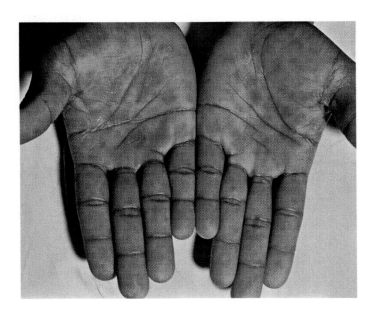

Figure 19–4. Secondary syphilis

Characteristic flat, slightly scaling lesions on palms. An almost pathognomonic sign.

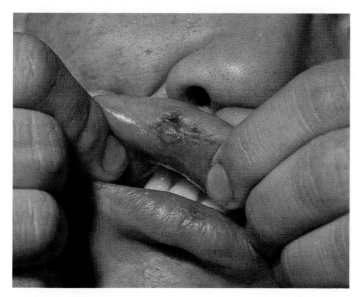

Figure 19–5.   Mucous patch of syphilis

Relatively inconspicuous painless eroded patch occurring during the spirochetemic phase of early syphilis. A highly infectious lesion.

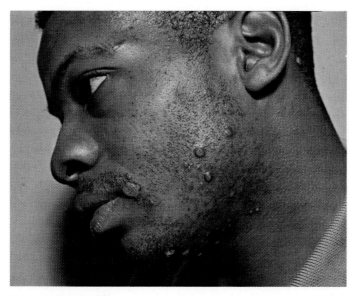

Figure 19–6.   Secondary syphilis

Slightly eroded papules occurring in late secondary syphilis. Spirochetes demonstrable in serum expressed from surface of papules. The lesions were quite firm. Temporary exacerbation of the lesions would be anticipated when penicillin is administered.

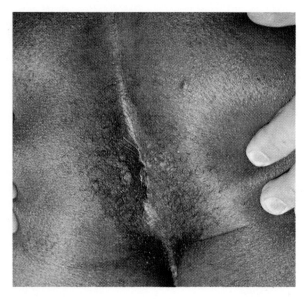

Figure 19–7. Secondary syphilis

Inconspicuous, slightly eroded, wart-like moist papules of perianal region. Diagnosis easily missed by the unwary.

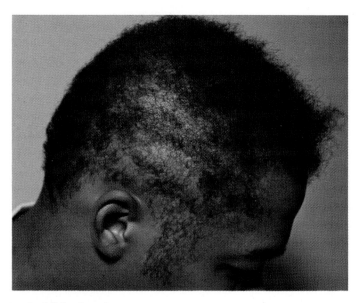

Figure 19–8. Syphilitic alopecia

Moth-eaten-appearing partial alopecia along sides of scalp in secondary syphilis. Hair regrows after treatment.

20

Parasitic Infestations and Diseases Caused by Arthropods

PARASITIC INFESTATIONS

The human skin is prey to an enormous number and variety of parasites. Those that are vectors of systemic infections are, of course, the most important. The remainder produce discomfort and disability principally through immediate and sequential reactions in the skin. Death may result from multiple insect bites, particularly from bees, wasps, yellow jackets, scorpions and hornets, because of massive introduction of toxic substances or because of anaphylactic shock. Such occurrences are not rare; insects probably surpass snakes in the frequency with which they produce fatal bite reactions.

The systemic infections that are transmitted by insect vectors include particularly trypanosomiasis, malaria, leishmaniasis, filariasis, onchocerciasis, loaiasis, Rocky Mountain spotted fever, plague, murine typhus, tularemia, epidemic typhus, scrub typhus and rickettsial pox. In addition, there are those parasitic infestations that primarily attack visceral organs. The enormous importance of these diseases in the medical, economic, agricultural and political lives of many parts of the world is difficult to appreciate fully unless one has observed them personally. With the rise of so-called primitive nations and the expansion of jet flights to and from them, the physician practicing in areas of good hygiene and public health control cannot safely remain indifferent to the possibility of the occurrence of "tropical" diseases in his daily practice.

Leishmaniasis

Three morphologically similar species of protozoa cause three distinct varieties of leishmaniasis.

1. Leishmania donovani (kala-azar, visceral leishmaniasis)
2. Leishmania tropica (Oriental sore, cutaneous leishmaniasis)
3. Leishmania braziliensis (mucocutaneous leishmaniasis, American leishmaniasis)

Cutaneous lesions vary from pigmented spots (as in late kala-azar) to granulomatous nodules containing a mass of reticuloendothelial cells and to the characteristic ulcer of Oriental sore. The latter lesion is prevalent in many tropical and subtropical areas of Asia, Europe, Africa, Central America and South America. The disease is most common in children. The infection is usually introduced by the bite of a parasitized *Phlebotomus* fly, and the incubation period varies from weeks to months.

The lesion appears at the site of inoculation as a slowly growing papule, usually on an exposed part, suggesting an itchy insect bite. Soon it becomes scaly, enlarges to form a firm round plaque or button and eventually ulcerates. Satellite papules may develop near by and evolve in the same manner. After a variable period of 2 to 12 months, the ulcers heal by granulation and scar formation; the latter are often sunken and deforming. Diagnosis is afforded by visualization of the parasites in smears from the margins of the ulcer base. The parasites may be cultured on Nicolle-Novy-MacNeal (NNM) medium. Intradermal injection of an appropriate leishmanial antigen evokes a tuberculin response.

Treatment is ordinarily infiltration with quinacrine or berberine sulfate. For numerous lesions and systemic infection, parenteral injections of sodium antimony gluconate are indicated. Secondary bacterial infection is common. Leishmaniasis confers a solid immunity.

Pinworm Infection (Oxyuriasis)

The chief dermatologic manifestation of this common, often familial, intestinal infestation is pruritus ani, usually nocturnal and extending to surrounding areas. The proper diagnosis in such itching may be easily overlooked. The eggs of *Enterobius vermicularis* may be recovered and demonstrated by applying strips of adhesive cellophane to the perianal area and anal orifice. The small round worms may be observed on toilet paper. Piperazine citrate or piperazine adipate, in doses of 65 mg. per kg. over a period of 1 week (maximum of 2 gm. daily) is an effective remedy, as is oxytetracycline. Thiabendazole 50 mg. per kg. divided into 2 doses is effective. All members of the family should be treated. It may be necessary to repeat this in 1 week.*

---

*Mullin, W., and Imperato, P.: Treatment of oxyuriasis with thiabendazole. Texas Rep. Biol. and Med. 27:615–621, 1969.

Hookworm Disease (Ground Itch, Uncinarial Dermatitis)

This disease, variously caused by *Necator americanus* and *Ancylostoma duodenale,* is widely distributed to all tropical and subtropical countries. The eggs, deposited in the soil in feces, hatch into larvae. Under conditions of heat and humidity, the infective larvae ascend to the ground surface and up any moist object — walls, trees, animals — for a maximum distance of about 10 inches. The parasites are thermotropic and bore through the skin of any animal indiscriminately, although they cannot survive in some "animal traps." In man the parasites reach the blood stream, are carried to the lungs and eventually reach their feeding and breeding grounds, the small intestine. The chief skin lesion of hookworm disease is a variable papular, papulovesicular or even bullous eruption at the site of penetration of the larvae, most commonly the feet. There may be an accompanying urticarial rash and swelling of the ankles. Secondary bacterial infection is common. The rash is not diagnostic but serves to arouse suspicion in "dew itch" country. The diagnosis is made by demonstration of eggs in the stool. Tetrachloroethylene is the treatment of choice.

Creeping Eruption

A number of parasites may produce the clinical picture of this disease. The causative parasites are hookworms of the genus *Ancylostoma* harbored in the intestines of dogs and cats. The most important species, *A. braziliense,* is found most frequently in the southeastern United States, Central America and many tropical areas.

Eggs are deposited in the ground in feces and develop into larvae under appropriate conditions of moisture, warmth and soil. Sandy areas are favorable, and the infestation occurs most frequently through contact with soil on beaches, in children's sandpiles and underneath raised cottages. The larvae penetrate the skin and crawl about in the epidermis or epidermodermal junction for months. They are unable, except rarely, to reach the intestine to complete their life cycle. Because of this limited capacity for parasitism in man, the infestation remains almost completely cutaneous. The larvae are almost a centimeter in length but are difficult to visualize because of uncertain localization and surrounding inflammation.

A transient papule, vesicle or patch of dermatitis usually develops at the point where the larva penetrates, ordinarily on some unprotected portion of the body, particularly the feet, buttocks, hands or face. The parasite may become actively migratory at once, but the incubation period may be weeks or months, possibly due to a combination of lethargy of the parasite and gradual development of sensitization to it. A thread-like line develops — reddish, slightly elevated, pruritic and 2 to 4 mm. in width. The route of advance of the parasite is erratic and unpredictable, with formation of a capricious pattern of loops, whorls and straight tracks. The rate of daily advance varies from a few millimeters to several centimeters, and the parasite may lie considerably beyond the site of visible inflammation, making localization difficult. With several parasites, the pattern of inflammation may be very bizarre and diffuse, commonly with bullae, crusts, excoriation and secondary infection. The mucous membranes of the nose, mouth and conjunctiva may be involved, but this is rare.

Diagnosis.   Creeping eruption is so distinctive in its morphologic pattern that it can hardly be confused with anything else. Biopsies performed in an effort to demonstrate the larva are so frequently futile as to be unjustified. In long-standing infestation, the secondary inflammatory changes may obscure the basic pattern considerably.

Treatment.   The standard treatment of creeping eruption is freezing of the skin with carbon dioxide snow or liquid nitrogen at a point just ahead of the extending burrow. With a single to a few well-defined burrows this is relatively simple and moderately effective. With many intertwining burrows, the most likely sites of freezing become very difficult to determine.

Thiabendazole, 50 mg. per kg. body weight in 2 divided doses administered weekly, has been shown to be effective in extensive creeping eruption, although gastrointestinal reactions and dizziness may limit its usefulness. Preliminary topical application of the 10 per cent solution formulated for oral administration should be tried (Harvey Blank). It is applied 4 times daily.

Onchocerciasis

This infestation, caused by *Onchocerca volvulus,* is commonplace in Africa and has a limited distribution in Mexico and Central America. It is transmitted by "buffalo" or "coffee" flies (genus *Simulium*). Adult worms may be found in nodules produced by the disease. The invasion is confined to connective tissue. Enormous numbers of microfilaria may be found in the corium, even in areas that appear grossly normal. Secondary changes of lichenification, erysipelas-like induration and eczematous reactions are seen. Elephantiasis is rare. The principal complication is ocular, in some regions blindness develops in some 30 per cent of patients, but it is practically absent in other areas. Microfilaria may be directly visualized in the anterior chamber on slit-lamp examination. The eventual changes are probably allergic in nature, consisting of low-grade chronic iritis and iridocyclitis. Superficial punctate keratitis is common.

Blindness results from corneal opacity or papillary occlusion. The treatment of choice is suramin (Naphuride), which may, however, produce troublesome Herxheimer reactions due to rapid killing of the parasites. Surgical excision of large nodules may be indicated.

Schistosomiasis

There are two types of human schistosomiasis: (1) a purely cutaneous affection (swimmer's itch) due to schistosomes, for which man is an abnormal host and (2) visceral schistosomiasis, a serious systemic disorder with inconsequential nondescript cutaneous manifestations, due to the human blood flukes, *Schistosoma mansoni, S. japonicum* and *S. haematobium*.

Cutaneous Schistosomiasis (Swimmer's Itch). This disease is produced by nonhuman schistosomes in birds and mammals and is noted following exposure of bathers to fresh water lakes, principally in the north central United States. Scattered outbreaks throughout the United States and Canada have been reported. Salt water areas are not exempt.

The schistosome enters the skin but does not penetrate further. A prickling or itching sensation develops, lasting from a few minutes to an hour while the schistosomes are entering. A transient erythema or whealing results, disappears and is then replaced after 10 to 15 hours by discrete, highly pruritic papules surrounded by a zone of erythema. Vesicles or vesicopustules develop a day or two later, subside within about a week and leave small pigmented spots. Following very heavy exposures, a confluent erythematous and edematous reaction may occur.

Not all persons swimming in infested waters develop swimmer's itch. These puzzling differences are apparently dependent on the degree to which the swimmer is sensitized to cercariae and the magnitude of the exposure. If the skin does not react upon first exposure, the cercariae are not sloughed out of the epidermis for some 2 weeks, during which time they serve to induce sensitization in susceptible persons. As sensitization increases, the reaction develops more rapidly and is more severe, with resultant rapid rejection of the organism.

The epidemiology of swimmer's itch is complex and intriguing. Bathing beaches are inhabited by snails that release cercariae during hot weather, particularly during July. Release is more profuse in the morning and during sudden warm spells of weather. The cercariae are less abundant in deep water, and waders in shallow water are more likely to be affected than are swimmers. Drying the skin promptly upon leaving the water furnishes some protection. The best means of prevention lies in killing off the snails, for which a number of methods are available.

Topical treatment with antipruritic shake lotions is ordinarily all that is required. In severe reactions, however, a short course of corticosteroid therapy may be justified.

Sea Bather's Eruption.   The cause of this disorder has not been established with certainty, although there is some evidence to indicate that it is due to marine cercariae. It is distinguished clinically from swimmer's itch in that (1) the lesions are predominantly in the bathing suit area, while swimmer's itch is on exposed portions; (2) it is limited to salt water; and (3) the lesions are predominantly wheals rather than vesicle-topped papules. The disease is seen on the Atlantic and Gulf Coasts of Florida and is sporadic and unpredictable. Palliative topical therapy is ordinarily all that is required.

SKIN DISEASES CAUSED BY ARTHROPODS

Every human being has suffered in varying degree from the bites of noxious insects. The number of insects capable of producing skin reactions is numerous, and the range of reactions is extremely varied. The insects involved include spiders, ticks, bees and wasps, fleas, mosquitoes, gnats, flies, bedbugs, chiggers, beetles and grain mites.

The reactions, both local and systemic, depend on two factors: (1) the injection of varying amounts of a substance that is toxic to all humans and (2) the production of a local or systemic allergic reaction depending on the degree of sensitivity of the individual who is bitten. This range of sensitivity is remarkable.

With most insects, excluding bees, wasps and ants, the actual bite produces no more than an evanescent tingling or a moderately painful sensation. Although, some individuals are insensitive, most people will develop a wheal at the site of the bite within a few minutes to hours. This reaction may be more marked, sometimes leading to a large bulla that may evolve into a slowly healing erosion or ulcer with residual hyperpigmentation sometimes leaving a scar. In some instances there may be swelling and erythema, even lymphangitis, highly suggestive of an acute bacterial infection. Occasionally, in some individuals who are extremely sensitive and who suffer multiple bites, anaphylactic symptoms may develop, although this is uncommon except in the case of hornet, bee and wasp stings.

In the case of some insects, particularly fleas, the reaction produced may be of the delayed tuberculin type. If some of the mouth parts of the insects are embedded, the reaction may progress to a persistent granulomatous nodule. We have observed many instances of histiocytoma, particularly in women, in which the original etiologic factor appeared to be an insect bite.

The degree of pruritus following insect bites is often very severe, and the urge to scratch almost irresistible. This results in varying degrees of eczematization, and secondary infection is common.

Determining the precise insect responsible for the bite is sometimes relatively easy, as with mosquitoes, ticks and chiggers. Residents of areas in which particular biting insects abound can usually point the finger at the responsible culprit.

From the purely clinical standpoint, there is little doubt that many individuals, after repeated exposure, become hyposensitive to the bite of a particular insect.

One common chronic skin syndrome results from the bite of fleas, namely papular urticaria. In view of several epidemiologic characteristics of this disease, which primarily affects children of disadvantaged economic groups, it is surprising that so many theories and controversies have developed as to the cause. Affected children develop itching papules during the summer months. The papules are distributed principally to the face, the extensor surfaces of the arms and the trunk, especially the shoulders. In the usual case no insect bite wheals are ever observed. Itching is intense, sufficient to interfere with sleep. Due to repeated scratching and rubbing, extensive lichenification and thickening of the skin often develop, and secondary bacterial infection is a constant threat.

In addition to the striking seasonal incidence of the disease, at least in temperate areas of the United States, a history may reveal that the dermatosis developed following a move into an older house, particularly one with a damp basement, or it may reveal that dogs or cats are present in the household. Bedbugs have also been incriminated as a source. Hospitalization ordinarily results in quite prompt subsidence of the itching, unless there are secondary factors involved.

Pyrethrum insect sprays are usually effective for the environmental control of fleas, bedbugs, gnats, flies and mosquitoes. Scabies and lice infestations are usually controlled with gamma benzene hexachloride (lindane, [Kwell]). The control of ticks, spiders, grain mites and beetles is more difficult and usually requires more potent insecticides such as Chlordane lindane, malathion or parathion. Great care should be exercised in the use of all insecticides, particularly if they are halogenated hydrocarbons, organic phosphates, phenoxyalkanoic acids or carbamates.

Certain other insects deserve brief mention in respect to the fairly characteristic syndromes that they may produce. Bees, wasps or ants produce a prompt burning pain at the time of the sting. This is followed by varying degrees of swelling and redness. Systemic reactions are dependent on the degree of sensitivity of the individual, and prompt treatment measures may be lifesaving, including the administration of adrenalin or intravenous hydrocortisone and the judicious use of a tourniquet if the bite is on an extremity. One insect prevalent in parts of the southern United States, namely, the fire ant, may produce many hundreds of individual bites that can produce a widespread local response in the skin.

The kissing-bug deserves mention. It can produce a very painful bite. Blister-beetles were a source of difficulty in South Vietnam, particularly for soldiers who were forced to sleep on the ground.

Diseases Caused by Mites

These mites (chiggers, red bugs, harvest mites) live in grasses, shrubs, vines and grain stems and are particularly prevalent in the southern United States during summer and fall. Chiggers should not be confused with the burrowing flea (jigger or chigoe). The chigger larvae attach themselves to the skin of man and other animals, partake of a leisurely blood meal and fall off when engorged. Farmers, hunters, golfers, picnickers, berry pickers and harvesters are frequently affected. Chiggers achieved considerable significance in military medicine when American troops were on maneuvers in the southern United States in 1940 to 1943.

The larva is hard to see, but it produces a degree of pruritus and an amount and persistence of reaction of quite remarkable proportions. Lesions are ordinarily most abundant on the legs above the shoes, on the thighs and at the belt line or other sites of pressure where the progress of the larvae is stopped. The papules form within a few hours, are extremely pruritic and often become nodular. The red mites may, at times, be seen in the center of the lesions, but they soon drop off. The pruritus persists for days and, sometimes, for weeks. Secondary eczematous "id" lesions may develop, sometimes as a rather extensive nummular dermatitis. Bits of chitin left in the skin may perpetuate the reaction, sometimes to the point of a foreign-body granuloma or a delayed histiocytoma.

Prevention of chigger bites is best achieved by wearing clothing that fits snugly at the ankles, wrists and neckline. Insect repellents are only moderately effective. Farmers favor painting a ring of iodine solution about the wrists and ankles, but this bit of rural medicine is not recommended with confidence. Some species of chiggers are of importance as vectors of tsutsugamushi fever.

Topical antipruritic preparations are useful in preventing scratching. If extensive inflammation occurs, oral steroid therapy is worthwhile because the trailing complications of chigger bites may be severe and disabling. In persons with marked sensitivity to chigger bites who face inevitable repeated exposures, an attempt to produce hyposensitization by a series of injections of extracts of the insect may be indicated.

Prevention of Insect Bites

A number of reasonably effective insect repellents are available commercially. None of them is completely satisfactory in spite of the intense study of a great many compounds during the second World War and since. They appear to vary considerably in their repellent effects on different insects, and some of them have cosmetic properties that some individuals find objectionable. Their duration of action is relatively short, i.e., from 4 to 8 hours. Frequent reapplication is therefore necessary.

Scabies

Following World War II there was a steady decline in the incidence of scabies and pediculosis. Since the early 1970's, however, there has been a remarkable rise in the number of cases worldwide. Scabies infestations in particular have become a very common disorder. Communal living, overcrowding and poor hygiene among some groups have contributed to this recrudescence.

The skin damage is inflicted principally by the female *Sarcoptes scabiei,* who excavates a burrow in the stratum corneum, lays her eggs and dies. The larvae emerge and moult and the females are fertilized. Without treatment, the cycle is continuously repeated, and severe scratch dermatitis and secondary infection are inevitable.

The alerting clinical signs of scabies are (a) the distribution of lesions and (b) the severity of the pruritus, particularly at night.

The distribution of lesions, primarily short linear burrows with varying degrees of inflammation that often obscure the primary lesion, extend to the flexor surface of the wrists, the interdigital spaces of the hands, the elbows, the anterior axillary folds, the buttocks and genitalia in men and the breast areola in women. The lesions are few in persons of good hygiene; they are much more numerous in infants and those who bathe infrequently. In infants, lesions may be seen on the face. In mental institutions for retarded children, failures in diagnosis, plus neglect, may lead to extensive crusted lesions that might arouse little suspicion of the basic condition.

The transmission of scabies is largely intrafamilial or venereal. Treatment is highly effective. Sulphur therapy is medical history. The preferred treatments include benzyl benzoate emulsion, 20 to 25 per cent, mono sulfiram 25 per cent and gamma benzene 1.0 per cent. All are available in proprietary form. One thorough application from the neck down is usually sufficient. The same clothing should be worn for 48 hours. Elaborate sterilizing of clothing, formerly in vogue, is unnecessary.

If severe eczematous secondary changes or bacterial infection are noted, topical or systemic corticosteroid therapy, or *systemic* antibiotic therapy may be indicated. In times past, many cases of glomerulonephritis were the sequelae of secondary streptococcal infection of scabies.

Pediculosis

There are three clinical types: capitis, corporis and pubis. The first two are similar morphologically but keep very closely to their respective areas of action. Pediculosis *(phthirus)* pubis principally involves the pubic and surrounding hair but may be found in the axillae, or even in the eyebrows and lashes.

All types of pediculosis are so uncommon in the United States that they have sunk below the horizon of diagnostic consideration. Nits should always be looked for with a lens in pyogenic infections of the scalp or in unexplained posterior cervical adenopathy. They are firmly adherent to the hair shaft. In pediculosis corporis, the lice (cooties of World War I) are seen principally in seams of clothing, rarely on body hairs. The lice of pediculosis pubis are quite fat and easily visible.

The experience of World War II dramatically demonstrated the effectiveness of DDT powder in preventing pediculosis. It was no problem, except in some returned prisoners of war. Today, however, gamma benzene hexachloride 1 per cent is the treatment of choice. It is available as Kwell, which should be used with caution, since it can penetrate human skin. Repeated and extensive application, especially in children, may produce neurotoxicity. In Kwell-resistant cases, 5 per cent DDT emulsion may be obtained by prescription for limited use.

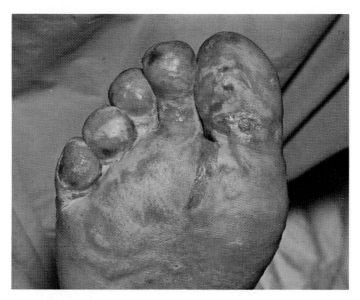

Figure 20–1.   Creeping eruption

Larva migrans of the sole of the foot, acquired from walking barefooted on moist ground contaminated with dog or cat feces. Freezing therapy would be impractical here, and topical or systemic thiabendazole is indicated for the larva migrans. Debridement, soaks and systemic antibiotics are indicated for the associated pyoderma.

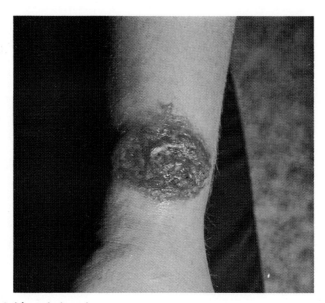

Figure 20–2.   Leishmaniasis cutis

Lesion observed in a Philadelphia college student who had recently been in Guatemala, Central America.

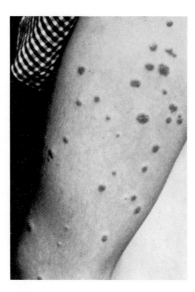

Figure 20–3.   Chigger bites

Reaction to chigger bites. The lesions are sometimes surrounded by a zone of erythema, suggesting a bacterial cellulitis. The itching is severe and persistent.

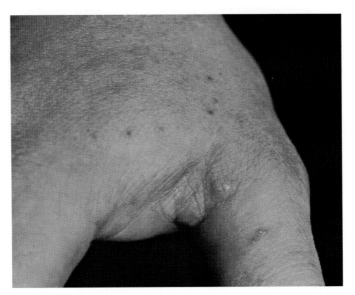

Figure 20–4.   Scabies

Characteristic interdigital burrows of scabies. If present for some time, the initial lesions are usually obscured by scratch dermatitis or secondary infection.

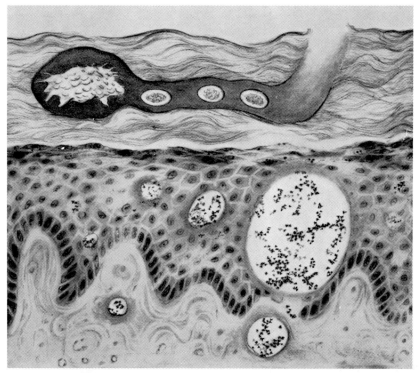

Figure 20–5. A scabetic burrow

The female Acarus, eggs and inflammatory reaction.

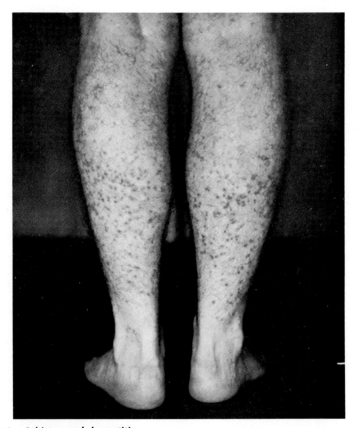

Figure 20–6. Schistosomal dermatitis

A sensitivity reaction to nonhuman schistosomes of birds and mammals, following bathing in fresh water lakes in north central U.S.A.

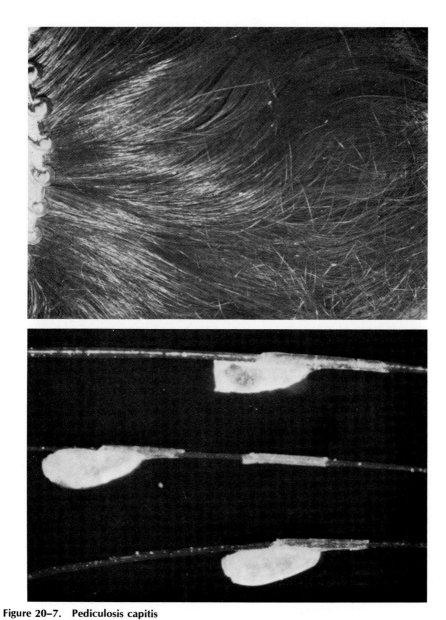

Figure 20–7.   Pediculosis capitis

The nits are adherent to the hair shaft and do not become dislodged easily, as do scales.

21 | Tumors of the Skin

The skin is an extremely common site for a wide variety of benign and malignant tumors. Because most of them are visible in their earliest stages, prompt recognition and eradication of them is possible in almost 100 per cent of cases. The most sobering exception to this rule is malignant melanoma.

The widely varying cellular derivation of tumors of the skin is outlined in Table 21–1. The following summary includes those tumors most likely to be encountered by primary care physicians, in whose hands a high proportion can be dealt with adequately. The primary critical goal in the management of any skin tumor is that the *first treatment shall be the last required.* Fortunately this is usually possible and constitutes a highly gratifying aspect of medical and surgical practice.

TABLE 21–1   ORIGINS OF TUMORS OF THE SKIN*

Tumors arising from the surface epidermis
Tumors arising from epidermal appendages
    Pilar (hair) structures
    Sebaceous glands
    Apocrine glands
    Eccrine sweat glands
Tumors arising from the melanocyte system
    From nevus cells
    Malignant melanoma
Tumors arising from melanocytes
    Epidermal
    Dermal
Tumors of mesodermal origin
    Tumors arising from connective tissue cells
    Vascular tumors
    Tumors arising from muscle, bone and fat cells
    Tumors arising from lymphoreticular cells
Cutaneous endometriosis
Visceral carcinoma metastatic to the skin

*Modified from Caro, W. A.: Tumors of the Skin. *In* Moschella, S. L., Pillsbury, D. M., and Hurley, H. J. (eds.) Dermatology, Vol. II, W. B. Saunders Co., Philadelphia, 1975.

Seborrheic Keratoses

Seborrheic keratosis represents a very common and completely benign tumor that ordinarily becomes evident at middle age or later. There is frequently a family history of such lesions. The initial appearance has aptly been likened to a blob of candle wax on the skin. Within months to years the lesion becomes darker and the surface more raised and verrucous. Some lesions become black and may be confused with malignant melanoma. The chief sites of involvement are the head, neck and trunk, although isolated lesions may occur elsewhere. Multiple seborrheic keratoses are commonly seen on the trunk. Fully developed lesions attain a diameter of 1 cm. or more, and coalescence of lesions may occur, producing large pigmented plaques.

Patients with seborrheic keratoses often seek medical advice for cosmetic reasons or, more commonly, because the lesion is assumed to be a pigmented mole. In most instances, simple inspection will indicate the true nature of the lesion and permit prompt, strong reassurance of the patient. In some lesions, a biopsy may be advisable for more certain differentiation. Aside from cosmetic reasons, seborrheic keratoses sometimes become bothersome because of irritation from clothing, hair clippers or combs. In many women of 50 years or older, these lesions occur as pedunculated "tags" on the neck.

Flat seborrheic keratoses are commonly seen on the faces of blacks in the form of small pigmented papules that develop at puberty.

Treatment.   The treatment of seborrheic keratoses is simple and effective, virtually without any significant complications. Since this is a wholly epidermal tumor, simple curettage is all that is necessary, using a sharp ring curette with preliminary lidocaine anesthesia. Bleeding may be stopped by *light* electrodesiccation, pressure, an absorbable gelatin sponge dressing (Gelfoam) or Monsel's solution. In thick horny lesions, curettage can be facilitated by preliminary light "cooking" with electrodesiccation. Should there be any question of the diagnosis, a biopsy specimen may be obtained with firm curettage or a 5 mm. punch. The above procedure should produce no more than moderate depigmentation. Full thickness excision is never indicated in a typical seborrheic keratosis.

In early superficial lesions, cryotherapy is a satisfactory method, particularly if multiple lesions are to be removed. Inquiry should be made regarding any keloidal tendency in the patient.

Basal Cell Epithelioma

This is the most common invasive tumor arising in the skin. Certain types are seen in childhood as the basal cell nevus syndrome, but these are very slowly invasive. Basal cell cancer is encountered frequently in persons of 40 years or older and is recognizable early on the basis of rather definite clinical characteristics. These include a somewhat translucent appearance, with telangiectatic vessels in the lesion and a central dell. A history of bleeding on slight trauma is ordinarily obtained. The tumors tend to appear in areas of most numerous sebaceous gland distribution and in regions most exposed to sunlight. They may be deeply pigmented, leading to confusion with melanoma and to excessive surgery.

The growth of basal cell epitheliomas is slow but inexorable. They may require years to reach a diameter of 1 cm. The chief threat of a basal cell epithelioma, insofar as life is concerned, is if it invades underlying soft tissue or bone or extends into an orifice such as the nose, ear or eye. Such invasions can only be due to prolonged neglect, however, and they are being seen with decreasing frequency. In some areas, notably behind the ears and in the nasal folds, the tumor may be of an "iceberg" type, much larger under the skin than is apparent at the surface.

Treatment.   The aim of treatment of basal cell epithelioma is to *remove every vestige of tumor with the initial procedure.* Confirmation of the diagnosis by biopsy is absolutely essential, and a specimen obtained by firm curettage, or the entire excised lesion, is adequate for this. The simplest method of removal of this type of epithelioma is curettage and electrocoagulation. This has distinct restrictions, however, and should be limited to small early lesions in which the possibility of lateral extension under the normal skin or significant downward growth is remote. In early lesions, the extent of the tumor can be quite accurately determined by curettage, the tumor itself being very friable and distinct from the normal surrounding skin.

Complete surgical excision is a highly acceptable method of removal of this type of tumor and permits microscopic determination of the completeness of removal. This is particularly desirable for lesions about the nose and the nasal folds, around the ears or on the eyelid margins.

X-ray therapy has often been used for treatment of basal cell epitheliomas, and such lesions are ordinarily quite radiosensitive. It has the disadvantage, however, of requiring several treatment sessions over a period of 2 weeks or so and is inevitably followed by some degree of x-ray atrophy, which may be particularly troublesome if the lesion is on an area of the skin that will be exposed to sunlight. It is not the treatment of choice for the usual early basal cell epithelioma.

In extensive, neglected basal cell epitheliomas, the Mohs chemotherapeutic technique may offer the only hope of cure. This consists of destruction of the tumor by successive applications of a zinc chloride paste, with histologic control. Training and experience with this technique are essential.

Actinic Keratoses

Senile (actinic) keratoses commonly result from repeated exposure to sunlight and from the passage of time. They are frequently noted in middle-aged sailors, sportsmen and farmers. The incidence is much higher in individuals who reside in areas with a high percentage of sunlight, such as the southwestern United States. They are rarely seen in blacks, and blondes and redheads are much more susceptible. Bald heads frequently develop multiple actinic keratoses. Actinic keratoses may be seen in young adults at times, and here the term "senile" is obviously inappropriate.

This type of keratosis, which is a definite precursor of squamous cell epithelioma, is characterized by a small area of reddish scaling, which then becomes elevated, with a grayish horny summit. Biopsy of such lesions ordinarily yields findings that may be diagnosed as "prickle cell epithelioma Grade 1/2." The progression and the number of actinic keratoses can be checked significantly by adequate precautions, including the wearing of a hat on exposure and the regular use of effective sunscreen preparations.

A considerable advance in the treatment of them has been achieved by the use of 5-fluorouracil, which has a specific effect on the keratotic and scaling areas without damaging the surrounding relatively normal skin. This is ordinarily applied in a concentration of 1 per cent in propylene glycol. Within 2 or 3 weeks, during which the preparation is applied once daily, the areas of actinic changes will become red and scaling and appear worse than previously. If application is continued for a week or two more, however, the affected areas frequently will recede and yield a surprisingly normal skin surface. In some patients, allergic sensitivity to 5-fluorouracil may develop and interdict further application.

Actinic keratoses that become prickle cell epitheliomas do not metastasize early unless the mucous membrane is involved. The situation is entirely different with keratoses of the lip, which may develop from exposure to sunlight or irritation from cigarettes or a hot pipe-stem. In such lesions prompt biopsy and adequate surgical excision are essential because early metastasis may occur.

Lesions that resemble actinic keratoses closely, but that are not in areas exposed to sunlight, may develop after the ingestion of arsenic, whether in the form of Fowler's solution therapeutically or from chronic exposure to sprays on vegetation. These may be associated with pigmentary disturbances of the trunk. The keratoses are most commonly seen on the palms. There is evidence that visceral malignancy may be more common in persons so affected.

Keratoacanthoma

Within the past several decades, another type of tumor has been recognized that has the microscopic characteristics of a low-grade squamous cell carcinoma but that is relatively noninvasive. It is usually self-involuting and does not metastasize. This is keratoacanthoma, which frequently appears quite suddenly, often in a warm environment. The lesion may attain a considerable size, e.g., 1 cm., rapidly and is character-ized by a rounded border with a depressed crusted center. The differentia-tion from a true squamous or prickle cell epithelioma with a potentiality of metastasis is sometimes difficult and depends on the history of sudden onset and the gross architecture of the lesion. Removal of the initial lesion is advisable in spite of the eventual tendency to spontaneous involution. Extension of the lesion to underlying tissues may occur, although uncom-monly.

Intraepidermal Carcinomas

Both basal and prickle cell epitheliomas may occur in situ, confined to the epidermis for many years but with a potentiality for sudden increased growth and proliferation. Some individuals develop multiple lesions of this type. They commonly occur on the trunk and may masquerade as a patch of seborrheic dermatitis or psoriasis. The gross appearance of such lesions, however, is unchanging and the progression relentless. On con-firmation of the diagnosis by biopsy, surgical excision is the treatment of choice. Small lesions may be destroyed by thorough freezing with liquid nitrogen. In some individuals with lesions of prickle cell epithelioma in situ, a history of ingestion of arsenic may be obtained.

Histiocytoma Cutis (Dermatofibroma)

This is a clinically highly distinctive tumor containing fibrous and vascular tissue. It occurs as a round, firm intracutaneous nodule, which when its edges are grasped, has the feel of a coin or button embedded in the skin. It is ordinarily about 1 cm. in diameter, flat, or slightly raised, and varies in color from grayish-brown to slightly yellowish. In some cases, a history of prior mild injury, e.g., an insect bite, may be ob-tained.

The lesions are most commonly seen on the lower legs or arms and are most frequent in women. Histiocytomas are often a source of much con-cern to the patient, but the clinical characteristics are so typical as to permit prompt reassurance. The lesion may involute slowly over a period of years. If removal is desired for cosmetic reasons, surgical excision is the only effective treatment.

Keloids and Hypertrophic Scars

Differentiation of keloids and hypertrophic scars is a commonly en-countered problem — one that often does not permit solution until many months have passed. A typical keloid, which may or may not develop after an injury or surgical trauma, becomes evident as a small, fairly firm nodule after a preceding wound (if any) has healed. As a rule, a hypertrophic scar becomes evident sooner. Absolute differentiation at this stage is rarely possible, but in patients with a familial or personal history of keloid and in black patients, the eventual development of a keloid is more likely.

Keloid undergoes a slow but inexorable growth, sometimes becoming a marked, lobulated mass, usually dark brown in color. The lesions are often symptomatic, responding to minor trauma or giving rise to spontaneous burning, itching and tingling. A hypertrophic scar reaches a maximum size and then remains stationary or flattens out over a period of months to years.

Prevention is the keynote in the management of keloid. Elective surgery should be considered with great circumspection in patients with a personal or familial history of keloid. Electrocoagulation or cautery destruction is strongly contraindicated. If there are signs of either a hypertrophic scar or keloid, an early trial of intralesional triamcinolone acetonide injection is justified, using an initial strength of 10 mg. per ml. In well-developed large keloids, a strength of 40 mg. per ml. may be needed, although infiltration may be difficult and seepage into surrounding normal skin may produce atrophy and depigmentation, usually reversible in time.

A fairly standard method of treatment of large keloids in the past was excision of the tumor at the base, followed by x-radiation. We have never observed an adequate response short of x-ray atrophy.

Epidermal Cysts

Superficial cysts of the skin are very common, occuring frequently in severe acne or arising spontaneously. They result from displaced epidermal cells or as a result of occlusion of pilosebaceous orifices. The trapped cells continue to produce keratin and sebum. They may remain relatively constant in size; uncommonly they may continue to enlarge to the size of a baseball. They may be very numerous in rare instances, as in the disease known as steatocystoma multiplex.

Treatment. Cysts sometimes disappear following inflammation, aided by the intracystic injection of triamcinolone acetonide (5 mg. per ml.). Severe spontaneous inflammation may produce involution by destruction of the cyst sac.

An annoying and cosmetically unacceptable feature of some cysts is the constant minute seepage of rancid contents.

Simple incision and extrusion of the contents of an epidermal cyst rarely produces a cure. The preferred treatment is incision and excision of the sac. If removal of the intact sac and its contents is accomplished, cure is assured.

A common type of epidermal cyst of the scalp is termed a *wen*. These sometimes give rise to slightly painful discomfort and some hair loss over the dome. In days when large hats and large hatpins were in vogue, unexpected firmness of fixation of the hat was accomplished by through and through piercing of a large wen.

Skin Lesions of Leukemia-Lymphoma

This group of diseases is so diverse in its clinical, hematologic and pathologic findings as to defy any brief summarization. A few words are in order, however, because certain cutaneous signs may be initial warnings of this group of malignant diseases.

Mycosis fungoides is the only lymphoma that begins with skin lesions and involves the lymph nodes and internal organs later. The first indication of the disease may be nondescript, dry, erythematous patches, which may look like psoriasis but do not quite conform to the characteristics of any common skin disease. The lesions have a tendency to come and go and are not diagnostic of mycosis fungoides histologically. This phase may last for many years or may be skipped entirely.

The disease then progresses to an infiltrative stage with variably thickened lesions that may be annular and that tend to come and go. The diagnosis may still not be confirmed by skin biopsy or by hematologic or bone marrow studies.

The tumor phase then follows, often with multiple ulcerated lesions. The diagnosis is now clearly apparent, clinically and histologically, and lymph node and visceral involvement may be expected.

The treatment of mycosis fungoides is complex. In the early phases much may be accomplished by corticosteroids applied topically or taken orally in small doses, by soft x-radiation in the Grenz range or by topical application of dilute nitrogen mustard solution. From this point on, one enters the complex field of modern cancer chemotherapy, best left to the experts.

The management of other less common skin and subcutaneous tumors listed in Table 21–1 consists essentially of histopathologic classification and, where indicated, removal by surgical, radiologic or chemotherapeutic methods. Consultation is frequently advisable.

Summary of Management.   The management of tumors of the skin may be summarized as follows:

1. Many tumors, e.g., warts, seborrheic keratosis, lipomas and intradermal pigmented nevi can be recognized as benign with reasonable assurance by the experienced eye.

2. If there is any doubt, biopsy should be carried out. In small lesions, biopsy should include the entire lesion. Accurate diagnosis and cure are thus obtained in a single procedure in a high percentage of cases.

3. A cardinal rule is not to remove any lesion that has the slightest potentiality for malignancy without having a biopsy performed.

4. With early recognition and adequate removal, the cure rate in cancer of the skin should approach 100 per cent. A notable exception to this is malignant melanoma, a highly untrustworthy and unpredictable tumor even in the most capable hands.

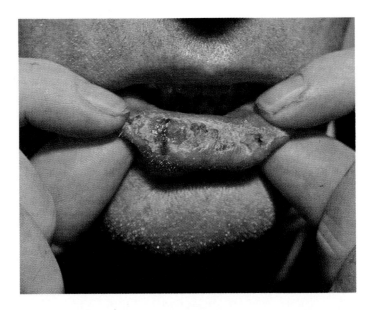

Figure 21–5. Actinic changes of lower lip

The lower lip is a common site of actinic changes and of chronic irritation from smoking or lip biting. The danger of early metastasis from a lesion of this type, if squamous cell cancer has developed, is considerable.

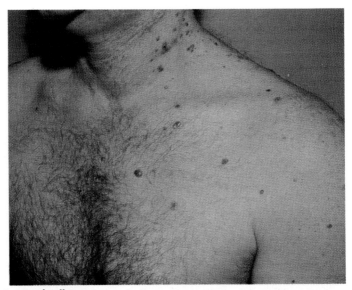

Figure 21–6. Basal cell nevus

This rather recently identified congenital syndrome is characterized by an autosomal dominant pattern, good penetrance, variable expression and skin lesions which are indistinguishable from adult basal cell cancer. The tumors, which are often mistaken for nevi in early childhood, increase in number and rate of growth at puberty. Actinic exposure is not an important etiologic agent. Dental cysts, punctate keratoses of the palms, milia, bifid ribs along with occasional disorders of the endocrine system, spine, eyes and central nervous system complete the syndrome.

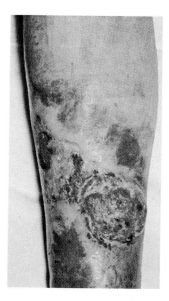

Figure 21–7.   Squamous cell cancer

The tumor developed in a burn scar on the lower leg. Chronic ulcers in such scars should be watched carefully for evidence of neoplastic changes.

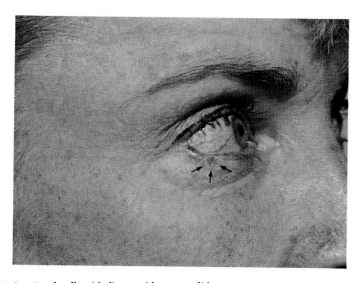

Figure 21–8.   Basal cell epithelioma of lower eyelid

Lesions of this type may masquerade as blepharitis unless carefully examined. Surgical excision indicated.

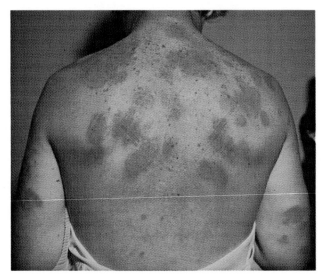

Figure 21–9.   "Id" reaction in acute myelogenous leukemia

These bizarre erythematous and slightly urticarial skin lesions developed early in the course of rapidly fatal acute myelogenous leukemia. Biopsy revealed no leukemic infiltrate in the skin.

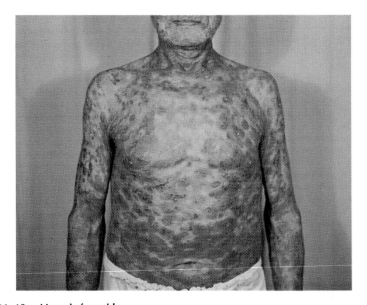

Figure 21–10.   Mycosis fungoides

Beginning tumorous phase of longstanding mycosis fungoides.

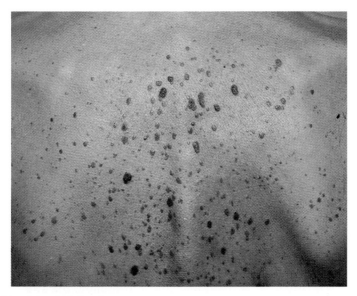

Figure 21–11.   Seborrheic keratoses

Very common superficial tumor, in varying shades of dirty-yellow to brown to black. Removal indicated only for cosmetic reason in lesions on exposed areas, or for mechanical reasons in lesions which become large and raised. Not precancerous.

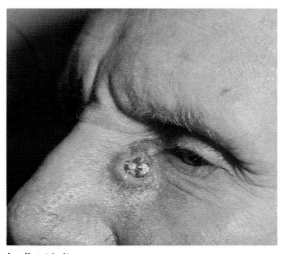

Figure 21–12.   Basal cell epithelioma

Typical lesion in a threatening location. Rolled border, central erosion. Note extension toward inner canthus. This lesion had been present for some three or four years; its earlier removal would have been a simple procedure.

22 | Hemangiomas

Benign angiomatous tumors, present at birth or developing shortly thereafter, are among the most common tumors of the skin. They are variously termed strawberry marks, cavernous angiomas and port-wine stains. A flat angioma occurring in the occipital region is so common as to be termed a "physiologic" birthmark. As a class, hemangiomas are not susceptible to any simple treatment, but fortunately, the strawberry mark involutes spontaneously in varying periods of time.

The terminology applied to angiomas in some large texts is cumbersome and confusing. There appears to be no classification that is satisfactory to clinician and pathologist alike. On the basis of different clinical characteristics and variations in prognosis, hemangiomas may be classified as follows.

Flat Macular Hemangiomas (Nevus Flammeus, Port-wine Stains)

These lesions are macular and ordinarily present full-blown at birth. They are common, particularly in the nuchal area, and appear as small patches about the eyelids and forehead. The latter lesions may become less conspicuous in time, probably due in part to the thickening and darkening of the epidermal layer as the infant grows older.

Port-wine angiomas may be so large and suffused as to be a decided cosmetic liability on exposed portions of the body. The color is intensified by crying or exertion and on exposure to heat and cold. Little hope for spontaneous fading can be offered, especially if the contrast with surrounding skin is marked.

Treatment. No effective method is available. Ionizing radiation, freezing, tattooing and various escharotics have all been tried and found wanting.

A variety of tinted creams for obscuring such lesions is available. Trials of them should be attempted if and when playmates of an affected child begin to note the lesion, often in a teasing or even jeering fashion. Young children often become surprisingly adept at applying such creams.

314

Obtaining a proper shade is important, and the professional aid of a skilled cosmetician is very helpful.

Immature (Strawberry) Hemangiomas

These lesions, developing or enlarging after birth, are very common. They are ordinarily small but sometimes involve sizeable areas. Almost all of them disappear spontaneously in time and they are not seen in adults. Opinions as to the treatment of such lesions vary widely; there are those who would treat almost all, and others who would treat almost none. The parents of children with such lesions often receive greatly conflicting advice.

Immature hemangiomas have the following distinctive features:

1. They often do not develop until after birth or, if present then, almost invariably enlarge during the first 6 months of life.

2. They are soft and compressible, blanching almost completely on pressure.

3. They are "immature" histologically, presenting poorly differentiated embryonal features, at times suggesting a neoplasm.

4. They may become ulcerated at times because of sclerosis and thrombosis rather than because of infection. This is more apt to occur in larger lesions than in smaller ones, commonly in lesions in the diaper region.

5. Spontaneous involution is heralded by patchy whiteness of the surface. If no erosion or ulceration occurs, the epidermis overlying the lesion remains intact. When the lesion finally shrinks flat, there may be hardly a trace. Involution is almost always well under way at the age of 2 years, often sooner, but no absolute prognosis can be given in this regard.

6. Hemorrhage from this type of hemangioma on injury, though much feared by parents, is usually of capillary type and easily controlled by pressure.

Treatment.   A wide variety of treatments have been used by many with no knowledge of the fact that hemangiomas of this type disppear spontaneously. Successive photographs at 3-month intervals are useful in judging progress.

For some 40 years the senior author (DMP) has followed the practice of not treating small, uncomplicated hemangiomas. This has been a rewarding experience in terms of final results and the absence of any regrettable sequelae. The only exceptions have been lesions that were threatening to undergo severe ulceration or that were occluding body orifices or an eye. Under such circumstances, *conservative* ionizing radiation therapy, *expertly* administered with carefully estimated depth doses and due regard for underlying structures, is possibly helpful. Doses of tumoricidal quantity, as were once administered, are unjustifiable, and the trend among therapists is one of increasing conservatism, some refusing to subject any infant to therapeutic ionizing radiation for a benign disease. The possibility of thyroid tumor developing decades later, following irradiation of the head and neck, must be considered.

Freezing with carbon dioxide snow is an old and simple method of treating small, immature hemangiomas. A piece of dry ice is cut to size and pressed firmly into the lesion for 5 to 15 seconds. A special apparatus (Kiddie) is available for making CO_2 sticks from ordinary cartridges. A bulla sometimes forms after the freezing. The *eventual cosmetic result* from this method is *less than satisfactory* because the normal epidermis overlying the angioma is destroyed, and a dead white scar results. It is not recommended. Liquid nitrogen is rapidly replacing carbon dioxide as the method of cryotherapy.

Small hemangiomas may be excised, but the irreducible risk of the general anesthetic ordinarily required in children must be considered in relation to a lesion of cosmetic significance only. With large raised angiomas, there may be an excess of skin when the angioma shrinks, and this may require excision for a good cosmetic result.

Systemic corticosteroids may be used to great advantage in patients with *extensive,* cosmetically mutilating, *immature* hemangiomas. Although several months of treatment using prednisone (2 mg./kg.) may be required, skeletal growth of the child is usually not significantly retarded. If involution of the hemangioma has not begun after three weeks of corticosteroid therapy, systemic therapy should be discontinued. Consultation with a pediatrician is usually desirable.

Mature Hemangiomas (Angioma Cavernosum)

A small percentage of hemangiomas are present in fully developed form at birth and do not subsequently enlarge except in relation to growth of the affected part. These lesions are composed of fully mature blood vessels and often contain numerous A-V shunts. Connective and fatty tissue components are often present, and the lesion may be relatively solid and not easily blanched on pressure. The color is often deeply violaceous, not red. *Mature hemangiomas do not involute spontaneously.*

Such lesions may be of more than cosmetic significance. Those affecting the trigeminal distribution (Sturge-Weber syndrome) may be associated with progressive calcifying intracranial lesions. An uncommon but severe complication of cavernous hemangioma is the sudden development of thrombocytopenia, usually associated with a sudden increase in the size of a single lesion. This may prove fatal (Kasabach-Merritt syndrome). Mature hemangiomas may bleed considerably from penetrating trauma. In large lesions on an extremity, there may be an associated overgrowth of bone and soft tissue. The Klippel-Trenaunay syndrome is distinctive, consisting of hemangioma, varicose veins, hypertrophy of soft tissue and bone and arteriovenous fistulas.

Treatment. There is no satisfactory method of treatment. Mature hemangiomas *are not radiosensitive,* and such therapy should not be tried. If the lesion is not on an exposed area, attempts at treatment are rarely justified. In lesions of the face, however, gross disfigurement may be the patient's lot, and plastic surgical removal may be justified.

"Senile" Angioma (Cherry Angioma)

These are small, slightly raised, bright red angiomas that commonly develop on the skin of persons over 50. They are largely found on the trunk. The lesions are not commonly more than 5 mm. in diameter. They appear to be of no significance, and removal is rarely indicated. If removal is desired, it may be done by surgical excision or bipolar electrocoagulation.

Lymphangioma

This malformation of the lymphatic system is a much less frequently encountered distant analogue of hemangioma. The most common type is lymphangioma circumscriptum, which is highly characteristic, appearing as a localized group of thin-walled translucent vesicles. Distributed chiefly to the proximal limbs, its appearance is so characteristic as to hardly be mistaken for anything else.

Of more importance is an associated occurrence of widespread cavernous lesions in areolar tissue, muscle, bone and elsewhere. They may appear as massive cystic lesions that show no tendency to spontaneous involution.

The only effective treatment for lymphangioma, if the lesion is accessible, is surgical excision. This is feasible only with superficial lesions, and recurrences are common because of difficulty in determining the precise extent of the process.

Venous Lakes

Venous lakes are greatly dilated, thin-walled venules without vascular proliferation, and are a type of senile angioma seen on the face and ears of elderly persons. The vermilion border of the lower lip is a common location, and because of a blue-black color, they sometimes arouse a suspicion of melanoma. The color disappears almost completely on compression. Removal for cosmetic reasons is easily accomplished by conservative electrocoagulation.

Arterial Spiders*

This is a fairly common type of lesion resulting from dilatation of superficial cutaneous arteries. There is a central arterial punctum, which may pulsate, with capillary extensions that give it a spidery appearance. Lesions may develop during pregnancy and are seen in association with hepatic cirrhosis, often in large numbers on the neck, face and anterior chest. If desired, they can be destroyed by coagulation of the central punctum.

Pyogenic Granuloma

Pyogenic granuloma is a capillary hemangioma that proliferates to a certain size, rarely to more than 1 cm. It is usually cherry red, but some lesions develop a darker, somewhat verrucous surface. The lesion is almost always solitary and often becomes lobular. The term pyogenic is a misnomer; the lesion is not primarily infectious in origin. It may sometimes follow a mild injury. The lesion is highly vascular and bleeds briskly on trauma or excision. With the latter, bipolar electrocoagulation is ordinarily necessary to control the bleeding.

---

*Bean, W. B.: Vascular Spiders and Related Lesions of the Skin. Charles C Thomas, Springfield, Ill., 1958.

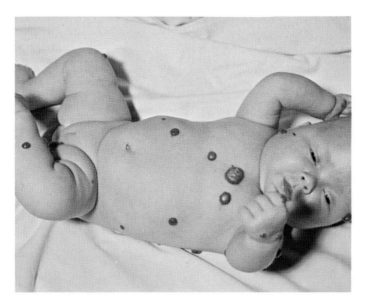

Figure 22–1.   Multiple immature angiomas

Multiple lesions in early infancy, enlarging after birth. (Patient of Dr. Matthew Olivo)

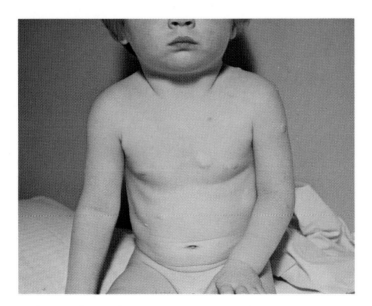

Figure 22–2.   Same patient as Figure 22–1

Spontaneous involution at age 27 months. The cosmetic result, while not perfect, was entirely acceptable.

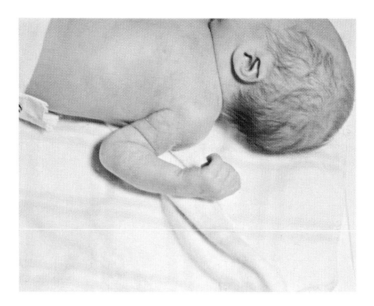

Figure 22–3.   Developing hemangioma at birth

This child showed only extensive telangiectatic vessels of the left upper trunk and arm at birth. Raised angiomatous lesions, however, soon appeared. Development and ulceration of raised vessels during the first 9 months of life is demonstrated in Figures 22–4 and 22–5.

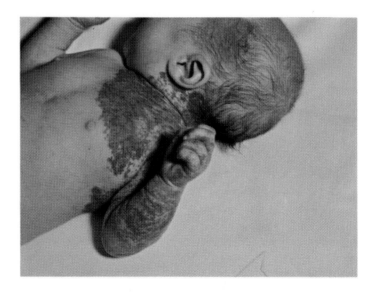

Figure 22–4.   Developing extensive angioma

Appearance at age 5 weeks.

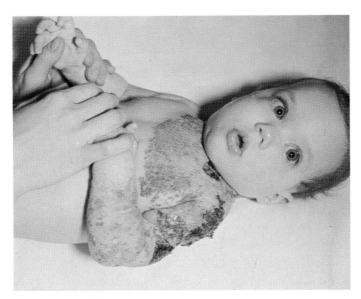

Figure 22–5.   Spontaneous ulceration of angioma

Extensive ulceration at 9 months. Note sclerotic whitening of nonulcerated areas. There were no local or systemic signs of infection. The angiomatous elements disappeared entirely, but marked scarring remained.

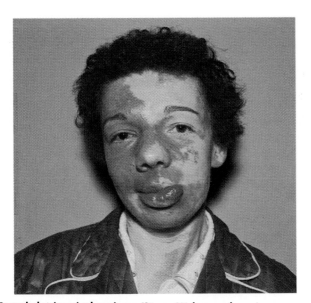

Figure 22–6.   Encephalotrigeminal angioma (Sturge-Weber syndrome)

In addition to the skin, there was involvement of the conjunctiva O.D. and calcification of the brain in the occipital region, with calcific debris throughout the convolutions. (Courtesy of Dr. Robert F. Dickey.)

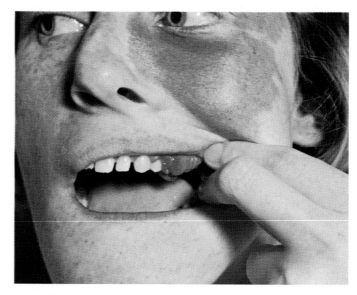

Figure 22–7.   Nevus flammeus with intraoral lesions

Intraoral angiomas may occur, but are not common.

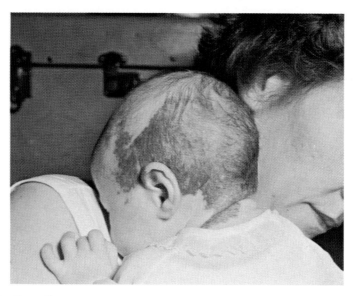

Figure 22–8.   Nevus flammeus

Extensive flat hemangioma with suggestion of some cavernous elements. Of little cosmetic significance because of almost complete eventual obscuring by hair.

23
Disorders of Pigmentation, Pigmented Moles and Alopecia

The amount and color of pigment in human skin obviously varies widely. Genetic and racial influences control this. Some disorders of pigmentation are inherited, e.g., albinism and a tendency to multiple pigmented moles. When the skin tans, melanin pigment is laid down by the melanocytes in the basal cells of the epidermis. The pigment granules gradually move toward the surface and are cast off. This is the mechanism of a fading tan. The presence of melanin in the skin is vital for protection against ultraviolet irradiation. Albinos, blondes and redheads are more vulnerable than brunettes and blacks, because they either cannot produce melanin at all or do so inadequately. Such individuals are much more susceptible to the development of skin cancer as a result of solar exposure through the years.

Vitiligo

This is a patchy loss of melanin pigment from the skin. The melanocytes, for reasons unknown, have lost their ability to form pigment. Initially the number of melanocytes is normal, but in long-standing disease they may disappear completely. A family history of vitiligo is often obtainable. It appears initially as oval or irregular patches of unpigmented skin that gradually enlarge. In the scalp, hairs may become depigmented. Associated alopecia areata is not uncommon. Although vitiligo is of no significance in respect to the general health of the patient, except in terms of possible primary pernicious anemia and thyroid disease, it can be extremely disfiguring and worrisome in dark-skinned persons. It is by no means uncommon.

The outlook for spontaneous remission in vitiligo is almost nil, and there is no truly satisfactory treatment. Methoxypsoralen 10 to 20 mg, by mouth, followed in 2 hours by cautiously increased exposures to sunlight or artificial ultraviolet light-A every other day may result in partial repigmentation in some patients. The outlook for total repigmentation in long-standing cases is guarded.

323

Hyperpigmentation

Many skin diseases and external stimuli or physical insults produce hyperpigmentation. The most common pigment is melanin, but other conditions produce other colors. These include the yellow color of jaundice, the reddish-brown colors of a variety of pigments derived from red cells, the characteristic blue-gray color of argyria, a somewhat similar color related to gold therapy, the yellow color of carotinemia and the bizarre pigmentation due to antimalarial therapy. The systemic conditions associated with hypermelanosis are legion. Perhaps the most common is the chloasmic pigmentation of the face associated with pregnancy or with oral contraceptive pills.

Treatment.   Reversal of melanosis of the skin is difficult. Excessive exposure to sunlight should be avoided. Two per cent hydroquinone creams are sometimes helpful but may be irritating. On the whole, the use of well-matched obscuring creams is probably best.

Pigmented Nevi (Moles)

Almost every adult has a few pigmented nevi, but they may number in the hundreds. The lesions are frequently of cosmetic significance. Moles are not all present at birth. They develop during childhood, often being transformed from flat brownish lesions to raised ones, which may or may not contain hair. This may be most marked at puberty. New moles may appear or old ones enlarge somewhat during pregnancy. Some moles disappear in old age.

The most important consideration in the examination of moles is the interpretation of changes that offer a possibility of malignant melanoma. Fortunately this does not occur prior to puberty. A dark slate-blue color is not necessarily a bad sign; it occurs when the melanin granules are deeper in the skin.

Small hairy pigmented moles that are raised above the surface and have a relatively even color offer no risk in respect to melanoma. Changes that should arouse suspicion in moles are:

1. The development of a ring of new pigment around the base.

2. The development of uneven pigmentation.

3. Sudden enlargement in a previously quiescent mole. In hairy moles, however, this may occur by reason of recurrent folliculitis and be of no significance.

4. Loss of hair in a mole.

5. Ulceration or bleeding in a mole. These, however, are late signs of malignancy.

Sometimes moles are present in the nail matrix and produce a striking line of pigment extending to the end of the nail plate. This is not uncommon in blacks, and offers little or no risk. When such a lesion appears suddenly in a white adult, however, it represents a truly untoward change. Nail avulsion and excision and biopsy of the mole are indicated.

If it is deemed necessary to do anything about a particular mole, surgical excision is the preferable method *with biopsy in every case*. If a melanoma is uncovered, it will be necessary to carry out a more extensive excision with grafting and, in some instances, to resect the regional lymph nodes.

Malignant Melanoma

Malignant melanoma is among the most vicious and unpredictable of the malignant neoplasms. Its onset is often insidious, and its growth variable. Because clinical diagnosis of this tumor is subject to a high degree of error, histopathologic changes must be interpreted by a pathologist with experience in its diagnosis. Criteria for judging the invasiveness of the tumor have been developed. Those of Clark, which are widely used, incorporate correlations between level of histologic invasion and prognosis.

Level I   All tumor cells above the basement membrane—"in situ."
Level II   Tumor cells present in the papillary dermis.
Level III Entire papillary dermis invaded.
Level IV   Invasion of reticular dermis.
Level V   Invasion of subcutaneous tissue.

With adequate excision, the prognosis in Level I tumors is excellent. It is only moderately less so in Level II. With Levels III and IV, the outlook is less sanguine. With Level V, the cause is probably lost, but chemotherapy, immunotherapy with BCG vaccine, and x-ray therapy may be tried.

It was formerly believed that excision of a malignant melanoma should be accompanied by wide dissection of regional lymph nodes where surgically feasible, even though the curative efficacy of such radical procedures remained unproven. There is still disagreement on the advisability of excision of regional lymph nodes, whether or not they appear involved; however, trends appear to favor a conservative approach.

Alopecia

Hair, particularly of the scalp, is an item of great concern to many individuals. Its growth is dependent on a wide variety of factors, particularly hormonal and genetic.

The most common aberration of hair growth is, of course, male pattern baldness. As is well known, there is often a family history of baldness among male members. Androgenic influences play a distinct role. When thinning of the hair begins, extending from the temporal region and affecting the top of the scalp in the late teens, the outlook for the development of significant baldness is almost foregone. It should be kept in mind that all males tend to lose some hair with age, although this may not be particularly apparent. For this reason, in males in their mid-20's who sustain some thinning of the hair, hope can be extended that they will not become significantly bald. There is no satisfactory method of prevention or treatment.

A considerable percentage of women are also subject to thinning of the hair in female pattern alopecia. It is frequently possible to obtain a history of thinning of the hair in other female members of the family. This affects only the frontal and vertex regions of the scalp. The growth on the sides and in the back proceeds normally.

The most spectacular type of loss of hair is seen in alopecia areata. In this condition there is a sudden dropping out of the hair in one or more small patches, or the loss may be much more extensive, sometimes affecting all the hairs of the body.

When alopecia areata develops to a limited extent in an adult, the outlook for regrowth without treatment is ordinarily good. When the disease begins in early childhood, even though there may be temporary regrowth, the outlook for cure is poor.

There is little question that corticosteroid therapy may stimulate hair growth in alopecia areata. This is not particularly effective in the form of liquids or creams, but small areas may be treated by the intradermal injection of triamcinolone suspension. Whether or not systemic corticosteroid therapy is justified in extensive alopecia areata is a matter of considerable discussion, since the disease being treated is of cosmetic significance only, and the assumption of unwanted physiologic effects from treatment is unjustified. Total alopecia has very severe psychic effects in some patients, however. The preferable treatment is the intramuscular injection of triamcinolone 40 mg. every 2 to 4 weeks. The success or failure of such treatment will ordinarily become evident within 3 to 4 months. The regrowth may be permanent, but more often there is a recurrence of the alopecia.

There are many other causes of alopecia, in particular, scar-producing conditions such as lupus erythematosus, burns and deep bacterial infections. Temporary loss may be noted following acute febrile illnesses that are not controlled promptly, as a result of the nervous habit of pulling the hair, in secondary syphilis and in ringworm infections.

REFERENCES

Clark, W. H., Jr., From, L., and Bernardino, E. A.: The histogenesis and biologic behavior of primary malignant melanomas of the skin. Cancer Res. 29:705, 1969.

Das Gupta, T. K.: Results of treatment of 269 patients with primary cutaneous melanoma: Five-year prospective study. Ann. Surg. 186:201–209, 1977.

Veronisi, U., et al.: (cooperative study). Inefficacy of immediate node dissection in stage I melanoma of the limbs. New Engl. J. Med. 297:627–630, 1977.

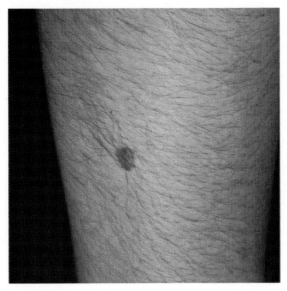

Figure 23–1. Pigmented nevus

Common "garden" variety of slightly raised, moderately hairy, pigmented intradermal nevus. The chance of untoward change in a lesion of this type in comparison to normal skin is probably little, if any. Routine excision is *not* indicated.

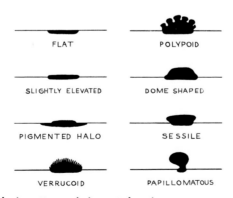

FLAT	POLYPOID
SLIGHTLY ELEVATED	DOME SHAPED
PIGMENTED HALO	SESSILE
VERRUCOID	PAPILLOMATOUS

Figure 23–2. Morphologic patterns of pigmented nevi

The presence of hair in any of these lesions is usually a comforting prognostic sign. The lesions in the left column are of types more liable to junction activity, with extension of a pigmented ring, changes in distribution of pigment and enlargement. (Shaffer, B.: Arch. Dermat. 72:120–132, 1955.)

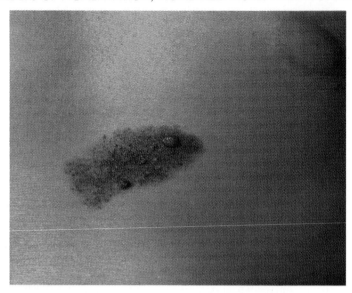

Figure 23–3.   Mixed pigmented nevus in child

Clinically this nevus shows varying elements and a tendency to extend peripherally. Excision advisable, preferably before puberty.

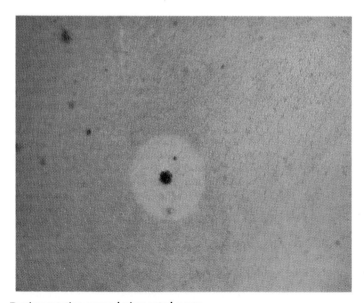

Figure 23–4.   Depigmentation around pigmented nevus

This is not an untoward sign. It is fairly common. It may be associated with nevus cell nevus, neural nevi, blue nevi and, uncommonly, malignant melanoma. The nevus itself may eventually disappear.

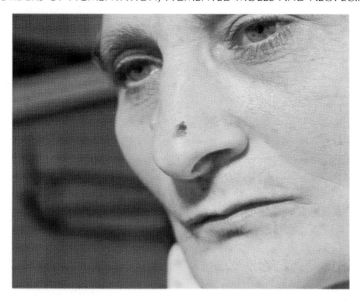

Figure 23–5.   Early melanoma

Clinical signs of conversion of nevus to active junction type and melanoma. Hairless, color change within lesion, extension of pigment.

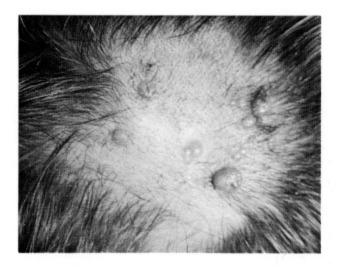

Figure 23–6.   Recurrent melanoma

Melanotic nodules in area of previously excised lesion. Active melanomas may produce little or no pigment. Five-year nonrecurrence of melanoma after excision is not certain evidence for cure; the tumor is a particularly unreliable and tricky one.

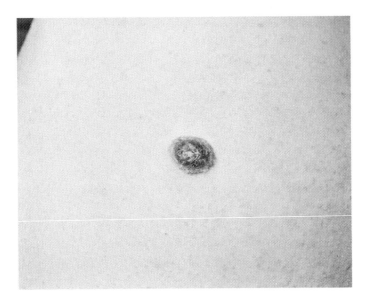

Figure 23–7.   Melanoma of buttock

This lesion shows the dark slate-blue color so commonly regarded as characteristic of melanoma. However, it is by no means always present and is seen in some benign lesions.

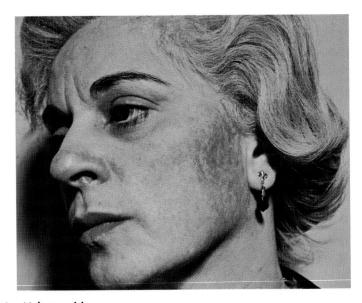

Figure 23–8.   Melasma of face

A variant of chloasma, which usually involves the forehead. May be related to cosmetics, pregnancy or contraceptive medication.

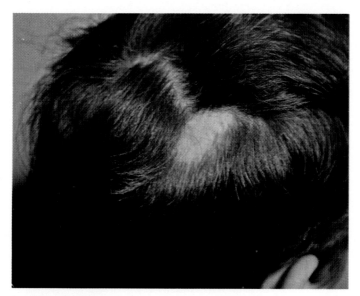

Figure 23–9. Alopecia areata

Single patch occurring in adult. Outlook for regrowth, with or without treatment, is good. Counter-irritants and ultraviolet therapy are useless. Topical corticosteroid may be helpful but often is not necessary.

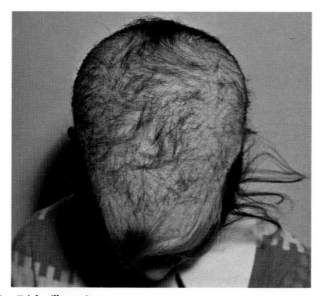

Figure 23–10. Trichotillomania

In less severe form, this habit tic of pulling hair is quite common in children. The clue to diagnosis is the absence of inflammation and the varying length of the remaining hairs.

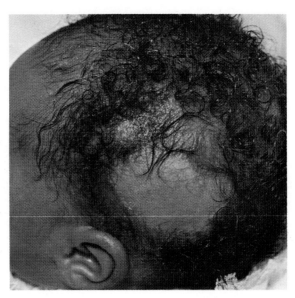

Figure 23–11.   Sebaceous nevus

The alopecia in the nevoid area is permanent. Lesion is not troublesome except after puberty when sebaceous glands become active and basal cell epitheliomas may develop. Odor and inflammation may be bothersome.

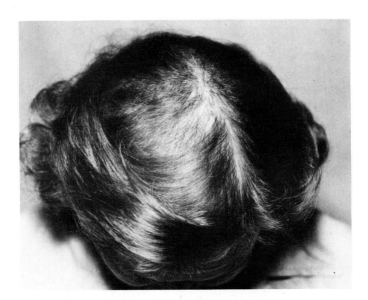

Figure 23–12.   Female pattern baldness

Hormone dependent, genetically determined alopecia occurs in both sexes. Typically, the crown of the head is most significantly involved. Post-partum hair loss and use of the birth control pill may hasten the development of significant alopecia in predisposed women.

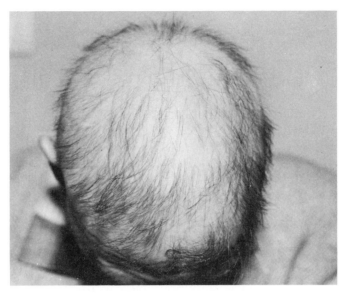

Figure 23–13.   Toxic alopecia

This child is on chemotherapy for a malignancy. Growing hairs are lost while resting hairs remain. Hair regrowth usually occurs following withdrawal of the toxic materials. Fulminating febrile illnesses may be associated with less dramatic examples of toxic alopecia.

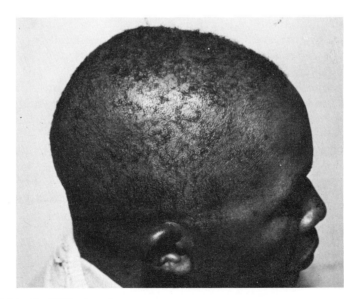

Figure 23–14.   Syphilitic alopecia

A patchy non-scarring loss of hair that primarily involves the occipital and temporal areas of the scalp is seen in secondary syphilis. Hair regrowth is prompt, following adequate treatment of the syphilitic infection.

24

Certain Diseases of the Oral Mucosa

The soft tissues of the mouth are subject to a considerable variety of lesions, some of them associated with diseases of the skin, others wholly oral.* In too many of these, the etiologic factors are obscure, and treatment is less than satisfactory. The conditions tend to be chronic; healing is interrupted by trauma to the soft oral tissues, rarely allowed a respite from talking, eating and drinking.

Canker sores (apthosis, aphthous stomatitis) commonly affect the soft tissues of the mouth. The precise cause is unknown and preventive measures and treatment are variably effective. First, a small erythematous papule appears, which soon erodes; an adherent greyish exudate then appears, surrounded by a thin inflamed halo. These painful lesions, 1 to 10 mm in size, rarely much larger, interfere with talking and eating. No systemic background is known. Although lesions generally occur irregularly, occasionally they may be almost unremitting. Rarely, the genitalia may be involved.

The pathogenesis of apthosis is obscure. Bacterial L-forms are suspect in many cases. Hypersensitivity to the normal bacterial flora of the mouth, as well as bacterial synergism, are also to be considered. To date, a viral etiology has not been demonstrated.

Aphthosis is usually easily differentiated from other erosive lesions, such as erythema multiforme, pemphigus and cyclic neutropenia. In extensive persistent lesions, however, differentiation from Behçet's syndrome may be difficult. The lesions usually run their course in 1 to 3 weeks without treatment. In extensive persistent lesions, however, the following may be tried:

1. Tetracycline, 250 mg. in 4 to 8 cc. of water, swished in the mouth several minutes, then swallowed. Repeat 2 or 3 times daily.

2. Corticosteroid applied topically as a cream several times daily or 5 mg. prednisolone in a small amount of water used as a mouthwash.

---

*The reader is referred to the excellent monograph, McCarthy, P. L., and Shklar, G.: Diseases of the Oral Mucosa. McGraw-Hill, New York, 1964.

3. To temporarily relieve discomfort, viscous lidocaine (Xylocaine) mouthwashes may be effective but make food tasteless.

4. In severe cases, systemic therapy with prednisone, 20 to 30 mg. daily for 1 week, or 1 or 2 intramuscular injections of triamcinolone acetonide (40 mg. in adults). Prolonged remissions may be achieved. Preventive measures are usually fruitless.

The following are representative of some of the more common and significant oral soft tissue disease, but it is far from a complete listing.

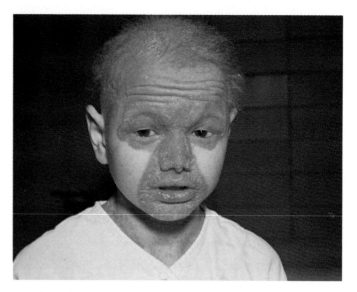

Figure 24–1.   Acrodermatitis enteropathica

Now thought to be a disease in which zinc is not properly absorbed or utilized, acrodermatitis enteropathica most commonly appears from 2 weeks to 20 months of age with equal frequency in males and females. The mouth, tongue, perioral area and hands and feet are typically involved. Clinically the lesions mimic severe moniliasis. Therapy with zinc completely controls the disease but should not exceed 45 mg. of elemental zinc per day (200 mg. of zinc sulfate).

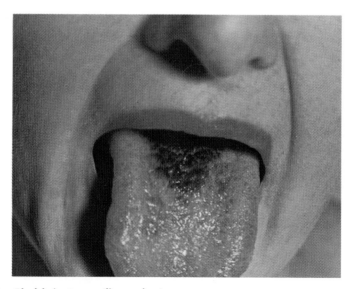

Figure 24–2.   Black hairy tongue (lingua nigra)

Brown to black pigmentation of the posterior dorsal surface of the tongue. In the uncommon "true" type there is marked elongation of the papillae. This discoloration is relatively frequent in patients on broad spectrum antibiotic therapy; it is produced primarily by bacteria and yeast that overgrow on the keratin of the papillae.

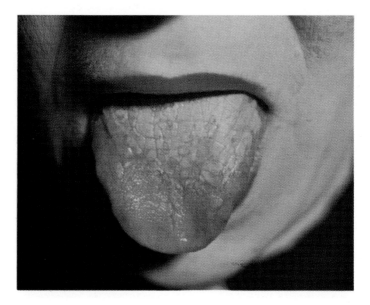

Figure 24–3.   Leukoplakia of tongue

Developing after lichen planus. Carries a real threat of eventual carcinoma.

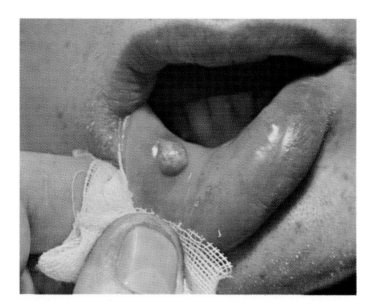

Figure 24–4.   Mucous cyst (mucocele)

Cyst possibly resulting from obstruction of mucous gland. Ordinarily curable by scissors excision of top of cyst and electrocoagulation of base. Complete excision sometimes necessary.

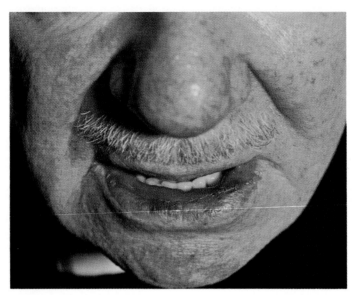

Figure 24–5. Cheilitis and pigmentation

Inflammation perpetuated by lip biting. Pigmentation of lower lip is common in older people. Venous lakes are the most common cause; these tend to blanch on pressure. If due to melanin, biopsy advisable.

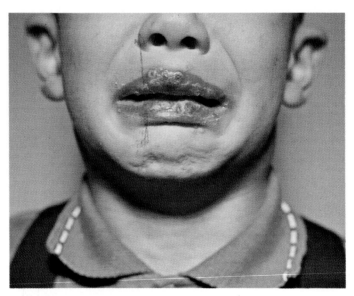

Figure 24–6. Primary herpes simplex (HVH) infection

Primary herpetic stomatitis may produce feeding problems in young and old alike. Therapy for relatively localized disease is supportive, since antiviral agents are toxic and relatively ineffective. Topical Xylocaine may provide some symptomatic relief enabling the patient to eat. The umbilicated vesicles and pustules seen here are clinically typical. Intranuclear inclusion bodies were identified on Tzanck smear. Herpes virus hominus serotype I was isolated.

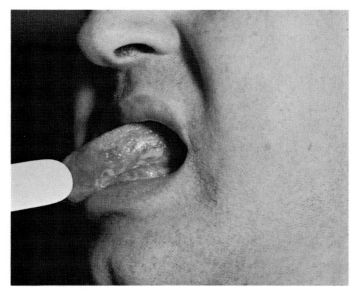

Figure 24–7. Pemphigus of tongue

This disease may originate in the mouth, without skin lesions. It is very painful. Diagnosis establishable by biopsy. Eating often uncomfortable and difficult.

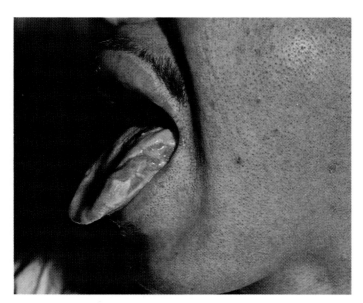

Figure 24–8. Ulceration from tongue biting

Biopsy revealed no tumor. A wide variety of oral lesions may be produced by tic biting. This patient was a diabetic.

Index

Page numbers in *italics* indicate material contained in figure or legend.

343